TABLE
— TO —
TRAIL

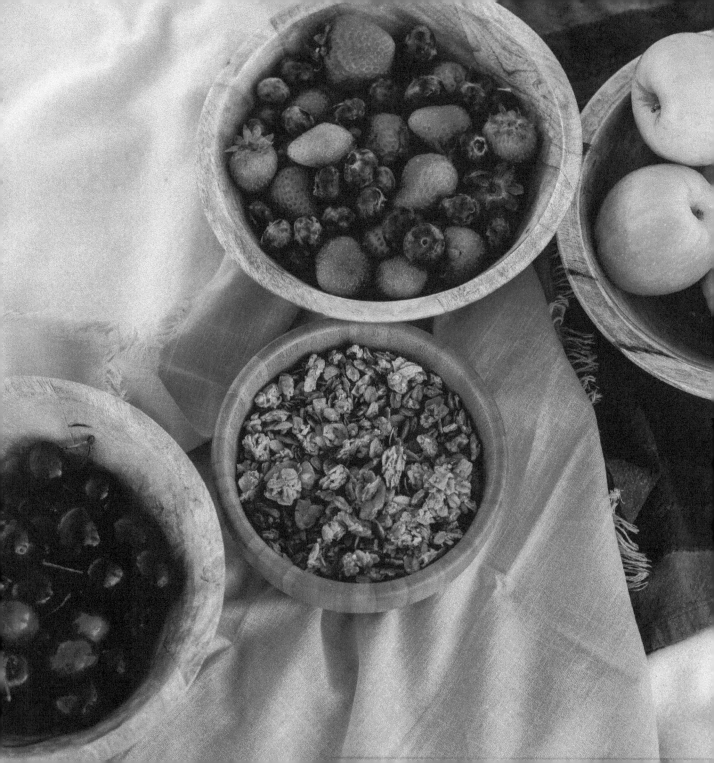

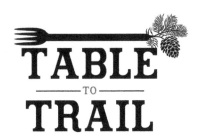

TABLE
— TO —
TRAIL

plant-based portable recipes for day hikers

MARTY COWAN

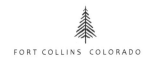

FORT COLLINS COLORADO

Table To Trail/ Marty Cowan. —1st ed.
ISBN 9780578728445

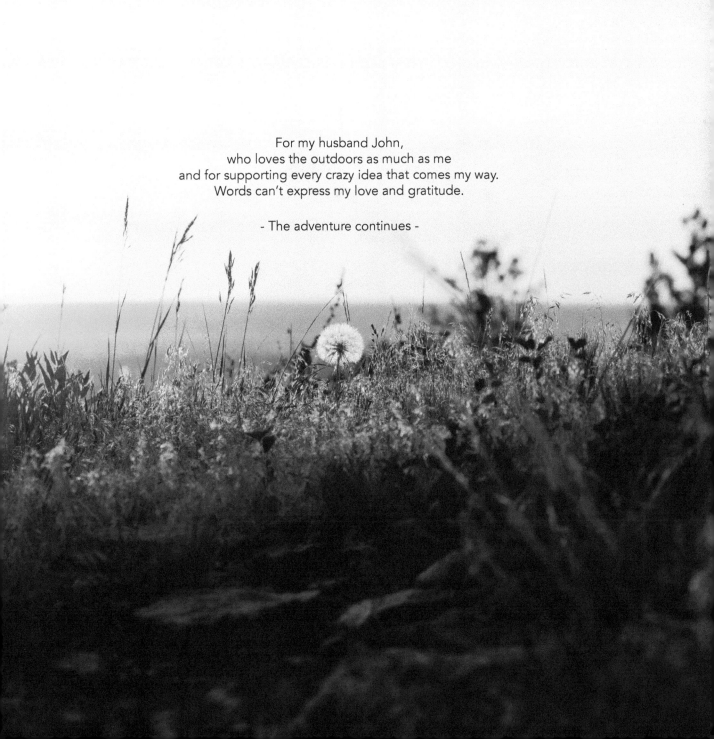

For my husband John,
who loves the outdoors as much as me
and for supporting every crazy idea that comes my way.
Words can't express my love and gratitude.

- The adventure continues -

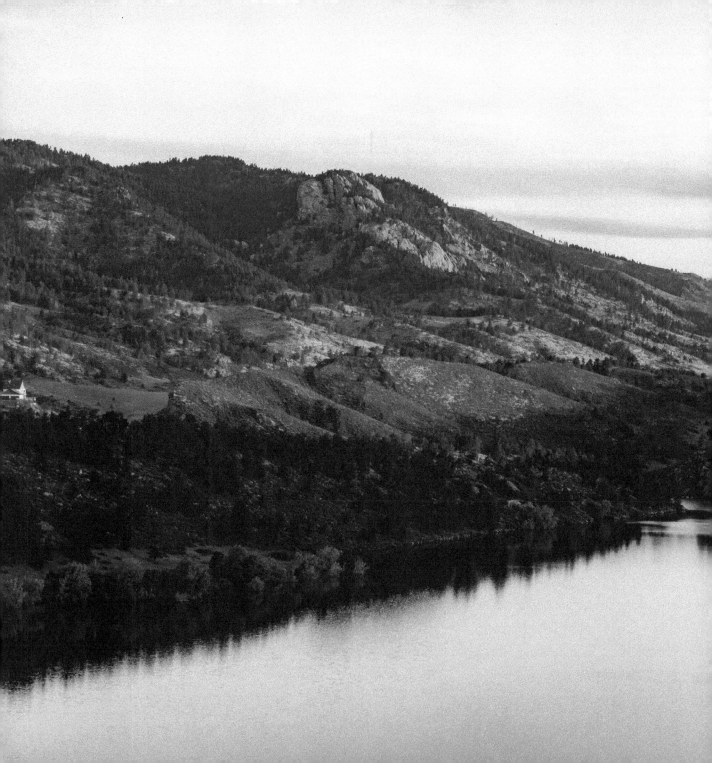

ACKNOWLEDGEMENTS

U.S. Forest Service, National Park Service and Larimer County Park Rangers

Colorado Search and Rescue Association

Colorado Trail Foundation

Protect Our Winters

Wild Bliss Photography of Fort Collins

Savory Spice Shop of Fort Collins

Whetstone Climbing of Fort Collins

Rescued Friends Animal Sanctuary

Kristin Hammond

Jody Jones

Merle and Marvella Crabb, the very best parents in the world

Clayton Cowan and Graham Cowan, we love you to the summit and back

WITH GRATITUDE FOR MY TRAIL SISTERS IN NATURE & IN LIFE
Lindsey Smith, Alex Franzen, Kelly Jancek, Lynn Johnson, Mikey Sullivan, Barb Grinter, Jill Jensen, Lisa Golicher, Heather Gossel, Kristen Castiglioni, Tricia Diehl, Brigette Douglass, Tania Hare, Andrea Rogers, Diana Vincent, Christina Kozisek, Lisa Hall, Lacey Steen, Chrissy Barker, Adrienne Gibson, Kristin Haber, Charity Chapman, Heidi Wallack, Rochelle Larson, The Real Housewives of Kechter Farm, Marsha Kaplan, Dee Satterfield, Kim Manfredi, Kerri Cooke, Laurie Sklar, Erica Chesnik, Savitha Enner, Stephanie Aldrich, Jamie Zimmerman, Mel Thompson, Vickie Walker, Annelies Antoinette, Eileen Robertson Hamra, Julie Reisler, Karen Saverino, Leslie Steiner, Donna Ripple, Denise Kelly, Polly Jessup, Jenny Sebor, Mimi Desta, Katie Egan, Jen Scicchitano, Adrienne Davidson, Britt Oergel, Nicole Brown, Kara Atkinson, Vicki LeBlanc, Randi Prager, Jen Hollander, Jen Butler, JJ Crabb, Stephanie Crabb, Meribel Crabb, Sue Cowan, Sherry Lyford, Dee Batis, Sarah Helland, Grace Helland, Dee Dee Dalton, Trish Rodriguez, Meghan Ryan, Stephanie Winter, and Laurie Yankowski.

WHAT'S A DAY HIKER?

A day hiker is a person who engages in a short-term hike during the daytime hours. This can take place in a park, designated natural area or a mountainous trail. These day excursions are generally local so that the hiker can enjoy the outdoors for a specified window of time, then return home. Hikes can range in distance and physical ability. There is something for nearly everyone to enjoy in nature.

Table To Trail food goes beyond tossing an energy bar into your backpack. Imagine a thoughtfully planned and prepared day hike meal enjoyed with the sights and sounds of the glorious outdoors. Find gratitude in the present moment of how fortunate you are to be able to explore the living natural world.

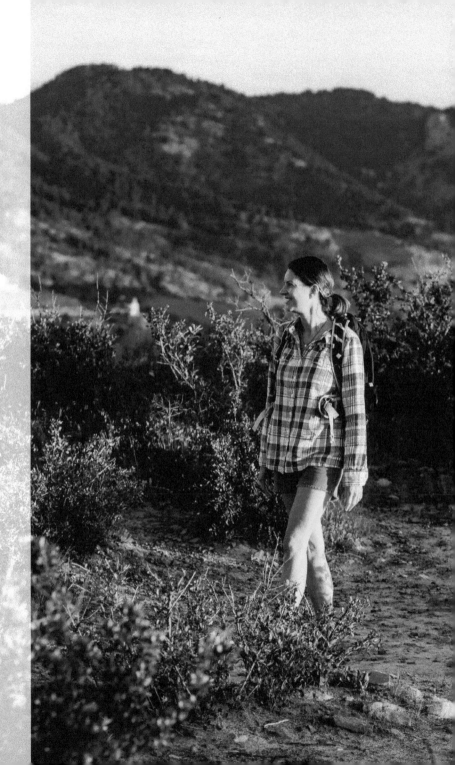

My dear nature-loving friends,

It's weird I don't remember my first hike or how I grew to love it with all of my soul. It happened slowly, and eventually turned into a need – like food, water, or air. Getting away from the stresses of life and retreating into the woods is like a physical, active meditation for the body and spirit. Taking notice of the surroundings – with all the amazing sights nature reminds us that we are here to enjoy the lush trees, fresh air and sunlight. It helps soothe our worries and frees us of the things that we allow in our lives that challenge our happiness.

By the time I was in my late 30s, I was exhausting myself with bad food and lack of exercise. Disease was on its way – it was just a matter of time. Like so many people I suffered from an overload of addictive instant gratification food, not enough exercise and a cycle of shame/starvation/overeating – this ruled my life for more than twenty years. One day I realized that the food I was eating and my lack of exercise was directly linked with my physical and emotional well being.

Our planet provides us with so many simple remedies to what ails us -- incredibly healthy, perfect whole foods and beautiful trails, parks and designated natural areas to explore. The outdoors are for everyone to enjoy. Take the time to see what's close by! When making the recipes in this book, add ingredients, take away ingredients – do what's best for your personal taste and specific health needs. Then pack it all up and take it out into nature.

Happy and healthy trails
and all my love,

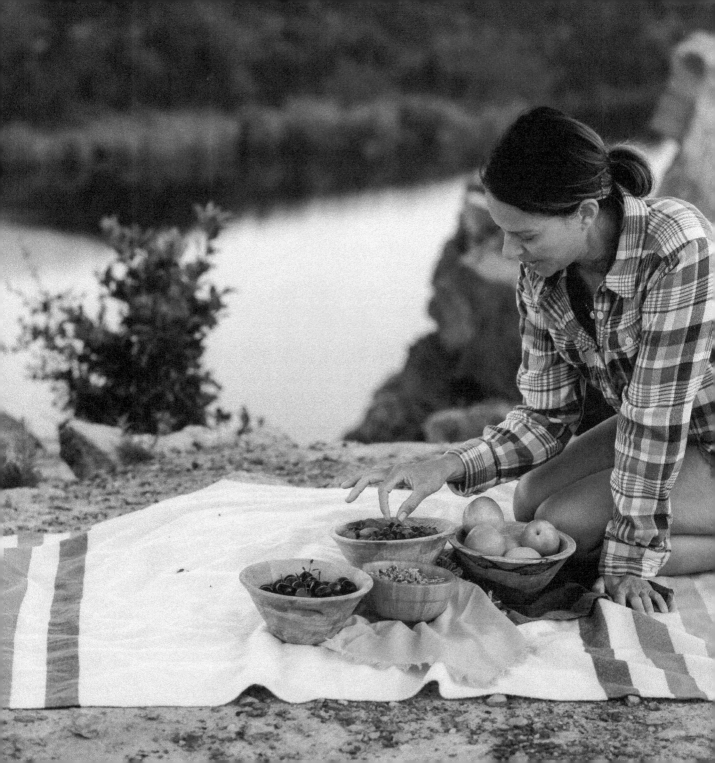

TABLE OF CONTENTS

GOOD STUFF that stocks the pantry and fridge is great to have on hand so you can prepare and cook a lot without a special trip to the store. The pantry items and equipment listed in this section are not mandatory, just suggestions for a well-rounded, plant-based kitchen. When it comes to equipment, don't worry if you don't have big-ticket items like a counter-top mixer – take it slow and decide what your specific needs are as you grow and develop in your kitchen. Take extra care to clean and thoughtfully arrange your pantry - an organized space greatly enhances the overall enjoyment of the cooking experience. Set aside a moment to be thankful for the bounty of what your kitchen has to offer you and your family each day.

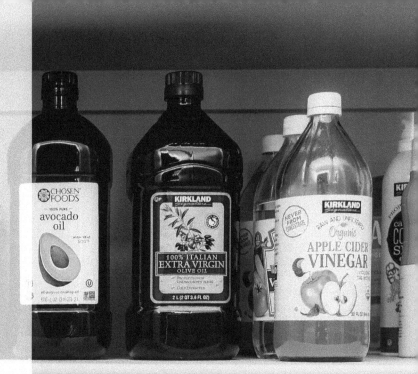

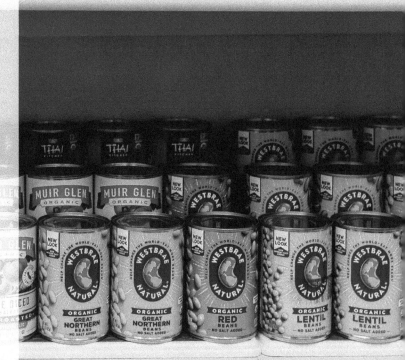

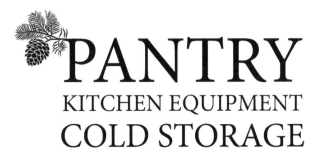

PANTRY
KITCHEN EQUIPMENT
COLD STORAGE

EQUIPMENT
Pots ranging from small to extra large
Mixing bowls ranging from small to extra large
Cast iron skillet
Small food processor
Large food processor
Manual chopper
Countertop mixer
Mandoline
Instant Pot
Rice cooker
Vegetable dicer
Julienne peeler
Vegetable peeler
Whisk
High power blender
Grater or zester
Chef's knife
Serrated bread knife
Paring knife
Mortar and pestle
Toothpicks
Skewers

BEANS/LEGUMES (canned/dried)
Black beans
Black-eyed peas
Garbanzo beans
Red lentils
Green lentils
Black beluga lentils
Yellow split peas
Mung beans
Pinto beans
Cannellini beans
Navy beans

GRAINS + PASTA
Brown rice
While basmati
Brown basmati
Wild rice blend
Pearled barley
Millet
Old-Fashioned rolled oats
Polenta
Quinoa (a seed, not a grain)
Spaghetti
Farfelle
Rotini
Orzo

FLOURS
All-Purpose flour (or GF)
Garbanzo flour
Coconut flour
Almond flour

NUTS + SEEDS
Sunflower seeds
Pepitas (shelled pumpkin seeds)
Sliced almonds
Whole almonds
Ground flaxseed (flaxseed meal)
Cashews
Peanuts
Walnuts
Pecans
Pine nuts
Hemp hearts
Chia seeds

FRUITS
Dried cranberries
Raisins
Dried banana chips
Pitted dates

SWEETENERS
Cane sugar
Brown sugar
Shredded coconut
Maple syrup
Agave nectar

OILS + VINEGARS
Olive oil
Coconut oil
Avocado oil
Vegetable oil
Cooking oil spray
Apple cider vinegar
White vinegar
Balsamic vinegar
Red wine vinegar

NUT BUTTERS
Peanut butter
Almond butter
Cashew butter

CANNED + MISCELLANEOUS
Diced tomatoes
Tomato paste
Tomato sauce
Fire-roasted tomatoes
Chipotle chilis in adobo sauce
Coconut milk
Vegetable broth
Nutritional yeast
Baking soda
Baking powder
Tahini
Liquid aminos, soy sauce or tamari

MILKS + BUTTERS (Cold Storage)
Oat
Almond
Soy
Nondairy butter

CONDIMENTS (Cold Storage)
Miso paste
Mustard
Ketchup
Nondairy mayonaise
Pickles
Pickled jalapeños

SPICES

Salt varieties (kosher, himalayan pink, sea, etc.)
Black (ground) and mixed whole peppercorns
Poppy seeds
Sesame seeds
Basil
Parsley
Oregano
Thyme
Marjoram
Tarragon
Dill
Rosemary
Bay leaves
Coriander
Ground sage
Ground thyme
Ground cumin
Paprika
Smoked paprika
Ground cayenne pepper
Ground ginger
Garlic powder
Onion powder
Chili powder
Turmeric
Ground mustard
Mustard seeds (yellow)
Mustard seeds (brown)
Cumin seeds
Caraway seeds
Fennel seeds
Cardamom seeds
Red pepper flakes
Cardamom pods
Berbere
Sumac
Za'atar
Curry powder
Garam Masala
Whole cloves
Allspice
Cinnamon

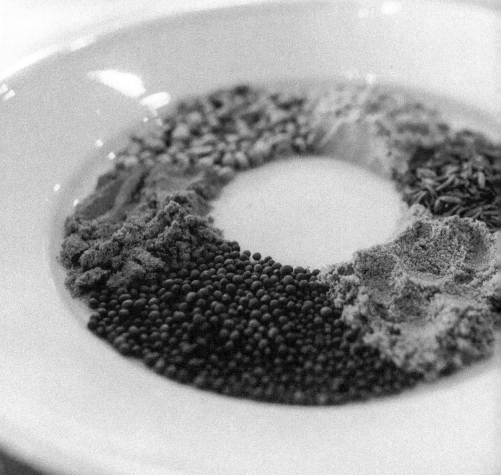

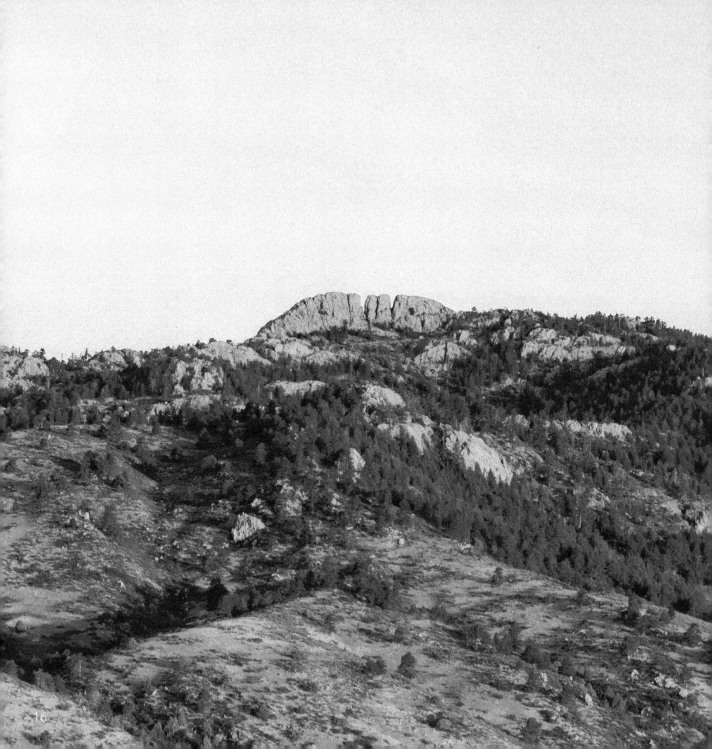

TRAIL PREP EQUIPMENT

PLANNING AND ORGANIZATION

TRAIL PREP: GET READY, HIKER!

Getting ready for the trail is one of my favorite things to do. Sorting gear and planning for my hike is always a happy activity – my preoccupation with the trail, nature and the meal is so exciting! Sometimes I even have have trouble sleeping the night before because I'm so giddy with anticipation. I love to savor the experience of packing my gear and the meals/snacks and setting out my hiking clothes. When I think of how lucky I am to have the time, the equipment and the means to get to the trail and back it provides so much comfort, joy and gratitude – the experience becomes sacred.

Hiking equipment doesn't need to be fancy. Use what you have and find out what your needs are as you go. An old backpack will do – check out secondhand stores and used outdoor recreational goods shops to see if there is something that doesn't break the bank. Another idea is posting on a neighborhood forum to see if anyone has an extra backpack or other gear they are not using. Many people may be willing to give it away. This is wonderful idea for new hikers to try equipment on the trail before committing to purchasing pricey outdoor gear. If or when you do choose to buy gear, make sure the retailer has a good return policy if it doesn't work the way you expect.

A way to organize your day hike is to establish trail facts go through the steps of your needs, depending on the particular hike.

DAY HIKE ORGANIZER

- How far away is the hike?

- Estimated timeframe

- Elevation gain

- Total distance

- Gear needed

- How much water is needed?

- How much food is needed?

- Who am I informing of my day hike plan?

- Is my vehicle filled with enough gas and current on maintenance?

EQUIPMENT AND SAFETY GEAR

Backpack with water bladder (or pack a water bottle)
First aid kit
Compass
Mylar blanket or emergency shelter
Weather-appropriate clothing (i.e. rain poncho, knit cap, gloves, etc.)
Phone with hiking app and trail destination downloaded
Satellite GPS messenger or PLB (personal locator beacon)
Bear spray
Bug spray
Tick repellant
Sunscreen
Knife or multi-tool
Matches/lighter
Headlamp
Hiking poles

Some of the gear listed above may not be applicable to your hike. Be sure to research the geographical area, weather and trail data of your destination. Read other hikers' reviews of the trail. Plan your hike so that you know a good stopping point for your meal, at what point to turn around and about how long you expect to be out. Let at least two others know where you are going and your estimated return time.

FOOD CONTAINERS

Before you get yourself into a buying frenzy, take a look at what you have that could work out on the trail. Before I had some of the more specialized gear for day hike meals, I used old containers that worked just fine. They may not keep food as cool or as warm as I would like, but when you are hungry and on the trail after a few miles (especially with significant elevation gain), hunger will kick in and the food will taste great no matter the temp. Many airtight containers will do. You will need to be the judge on what will fit into your backpack, and what food will travel best. For instance, I would put soup in an insulated container, because of the high liquid content. A standard airtight container for a dish with mainly grains would likely travel well in your backpack. And put your containers in a bag (insulated or a recycled grocery store bag) with utensils and napkins so that everything is all in one place. Experience what you have on hand and decide for yourself what is truly worth buying.

MULTI-TIER CONTAINERS
There are several varieties on the market for three, four and five-tier containers. Many are insulated to keep the cold stuff cold, and the hot stuff hot (or warm), even when stacked. In the containers, the elements of your meal are stacked and latched for easy transport – and can go right to the sink when you arrive home for cleaning and reuse.

INSULATED CONTAINERS
Try one of these for any meals or snacks you prepare - especially if they are heavier on the liquid. Also, the insulated container will keep the temperature more consistent.

UTENSILS
Always have set of reusable utensils in your pack. Varieties can include bamboo (or other products made of natural materials) or light stainless steel.

NAPKINS
A couple of cloth napkins pack well, and – unlike paper products – trees are spared. When I unpack, the cloth napkins go right from the backpack to the laundry room to be washed. Then they are ready to go on another adventure!

FIND A SPOT TO DINE ON THE TRAIL
I love to use the various large rocks/boulders on the trail as my table for my meal. A log can work as well – pick any spot that looks appealing! Let the trail help you decide on a good spot to stop and nosh. Bring a few large cloth dinner napkins to serve as a tablecloth. Enjoy the process of setting up your meal and savor each bite. Observe your surroundings, breathe in the fresh air. Feel the joy of being able to exercise while immersed in nature – then the pleasure of a delicious and thoughtfully prepared meal.

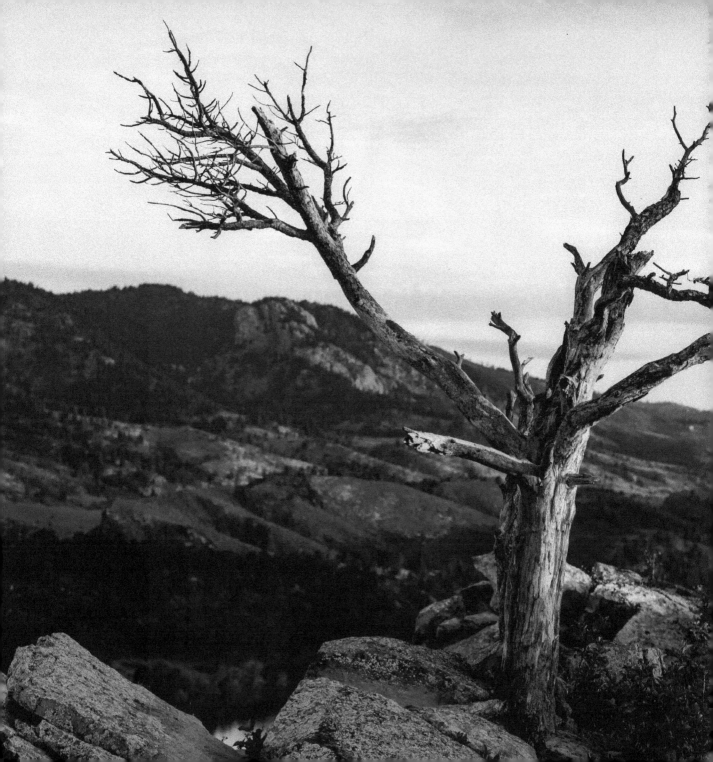

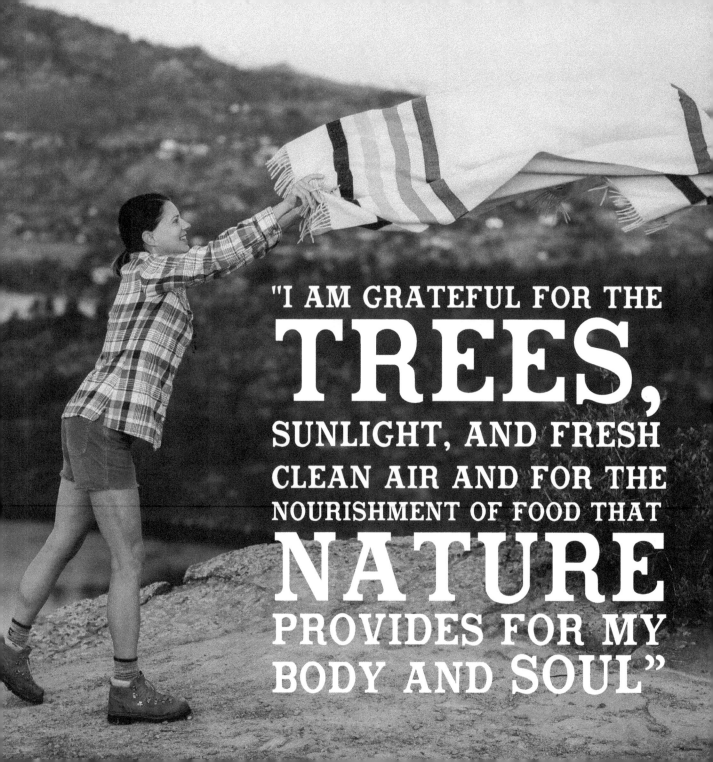

"I AM GRATEFUL FOR THE **TREES,** SUNLIGHT, AND FRESH CLEAN AIR AND FOR THE NOURISHMENT OF FOOD THAT **NATURE** PROVIDES FOR MY BODY AND **SOUL**"

FIND YOUR LOCAL TRAILS, NATURAL AREAS AND PARKS

Locate where you live on a map. Take note of how many hiking trails, designated natural areas and parks exist within a 25-mile radius. Write down the ones that pique your interest. Maybe there are ones that you have never even heard of before. You can also extend way beyond your search area to what I call "dream hikes." These are trails that are farther away – some may even require extra planning and travel.

Ask yourself, how much time do I have? Begin with the travel time to and from the hike. Then add to it how much hiking time you have. This will determine mileage and any stops for food or breaks.

What will I bring to eat? What you are in the mood for is key, and also the time of day can determine what you bring to nosh on the trail.

How much water? Climate conditions will be a factor. Overestimating on the water is a good idea, especially if you have a four-legged buddy joining you on your hike.

I want to explore the following 5 trails by _____/_____:

_____

_____

_____

_____

_____

TRAIL MANTRA

A wonderful way to begin your time in nature is to center yourself – take a moment to slow down and breathe. I like to find a grouping of words that are meaningful and represent how I feel about nature. You can think of your own mantra to use each time you visit a trail or natural area, something simple and easy to remember. Start your hike with this personal mantra. Repeat it out loud or to yourself over and over. Write your first trail mantra here – maybe it will stay the same or evolve over time.

_____

_____

_____

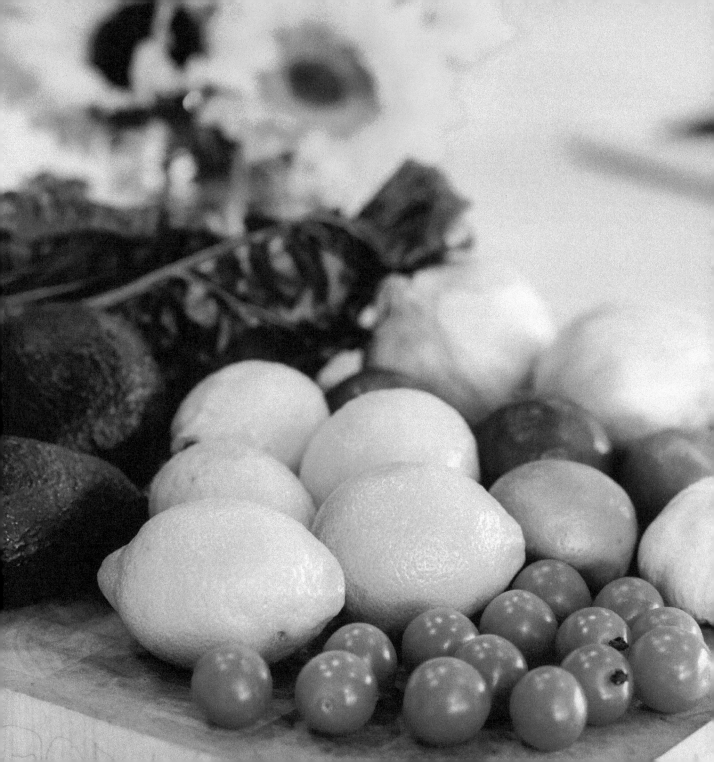

RECIPES

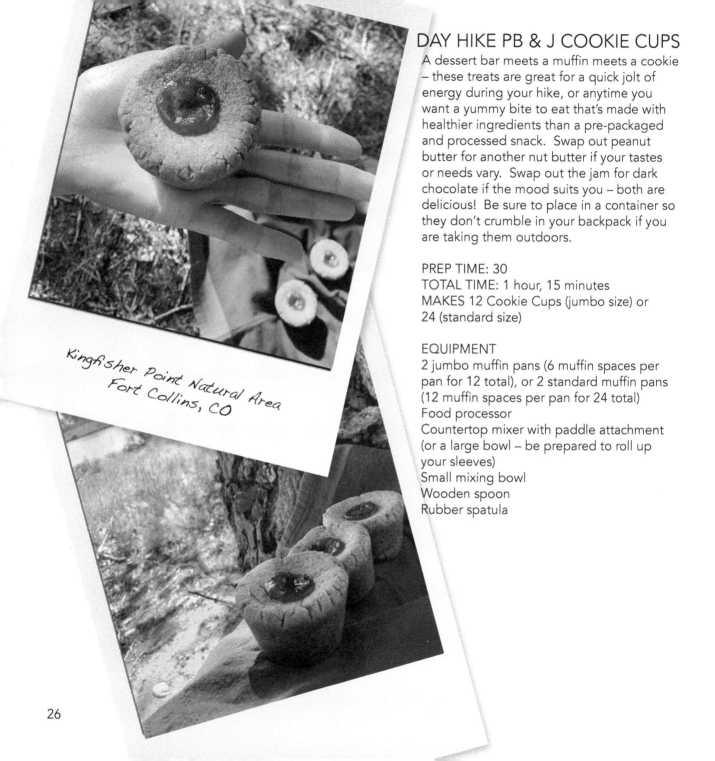

DAY HIKE PB & J COOKIE CUPS

A dessert bar meets a muffin meets a cookie – these treats are great for a quick jolt of energy during your hike, or anytime you want a yummy bite to eat that's made with healthier ingredients than a pre-packaged and processed snack. Swap out peanut butter for another nut butter if your tastes or needs vary. Swap out the jam for dark chocolate if the mood suits you – both are delicious! Be sure to place in a container so they don't crumble in your backpack if you are taking them outdoors.

PREP TIME: 30
TOTAL TIME: 1 hour, 15 minutes
MAKES 12 Cookie Cups (jumbo size) or 24 (standard size)

EQUIPMENT
2 jumbo muffin pans (6 muffin spaces per pan for 12 total), or 2 standard muffin pans (12 muffin spaces per pan for 24 total)
Food processor
Countertop mixer with paddle attachment (or a large bowl – be prepared to roll up your sleeves)
Small mixing bowl
Wooden spoon
Rubber spatula

Kingfisher Point Natural Area
Fort Collins, CO

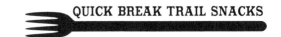

INGREDIENTS
Spray oil (for muffin pans)
Egg replacer (recipe below)
1 ½ C. old fashioned rolled oats
1 ½ C. all-purpose flour
1 tsp. baking powder
1 tsp. baking soda
1½ tsp. salt
1 C. (2 sticks) unsalted nondairy butter (set out from the fridge for 1-2 hours)
1 C. sugar
½ C. brown sugar
1 tsp. pure vanilla extract
2 C. creamy organic peanut butter (or other nut butter of your choice)
1 C. strawberry jam OR ½ C. dark chocolate chips

EGG REPLACER
2 TBS. ground flaxseed (also called flaxseed meal)
6 TBS. water
Put ingredients in the small bowl, stir and set aside.

DIRECTIONS
Preheat the oven to 350°. Grease the muffin cup pans with the spray oil and set aside. In the food processor, add the oats and blend for 1-2 minutes until smooth and powdery. Add the flour, salt, baking powder and baking soda. Pulse a few times then set aside.

In the bowl of the countertop mixer, blend the butter and sugars on a medium-low setting, about a minute, scraping the edges with a spatula as you mix. Give the water and ground flaxseed seed mixture one more stir and then add to the butter and sugar. Mix for about 20 seconds on low. Add the vanilla and nut butter and mix until blended at a low speed, about two minutes. Add the flour mixture to the bowl about ½ cup at a time on medium-low speed, scraping the edges as you go. When all the flour is mixed, turn off the mixer. Measure ½ cup of the dough for jumbo sized cookie cups, or ¼ cup for standard size, roll into a ball and place in the muffin pan. After you finish with all 12 (or 24), press each dough ball down into the pan evenly. Turn the wooden spoon upside down and make an indent for the jam or chocolate chips – or use your fingers to create the pocket. If you are using jam, fill each indent fully with jam, about a tablespoon each. If you are using chocolate chips, fill the indent with the chocolate chips. Place muffins in the oven for 25 minutes (for the standard size), 30 minutes (for the jumbo size) – test with a skewer to make sure the batter has fully cooked. When ready, take the cookie cups out of the oven and let them cool completely. Pop them out to enjoy right away, or store in an airtight container. These also freeze well (for up to a month) – just allow about an hour to thaw before enjoying.

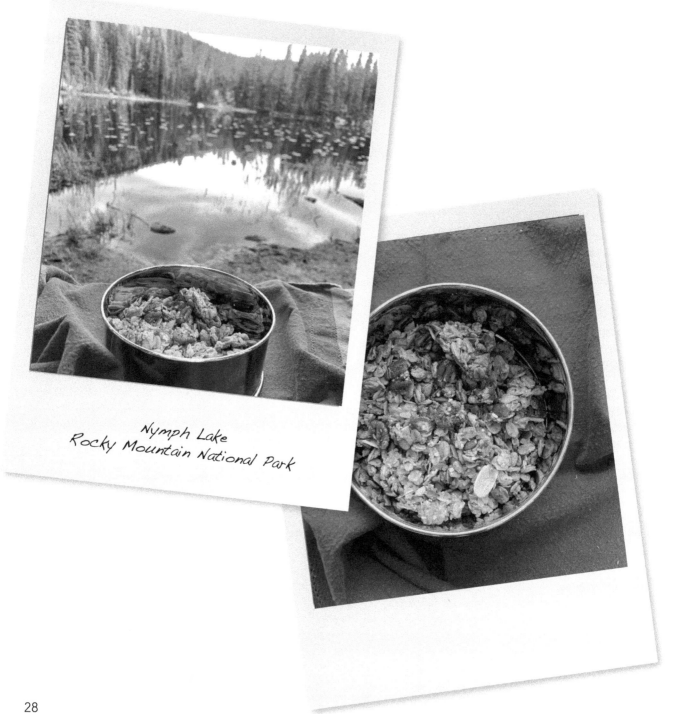

Nymph Lake
Rocky Mountain National Park

JOHN'S FAVORITE GRANOLA

This baked granola is crunchy, lightly sweet and perfect for a trail break or a quick breakfast on your way out the door. My husband puts it on his yogurt and requested after his first try, "no more store-bought granola, please," which makes me happy, because I love it, too. For a hike I put this in an airtight, insulated container and pop it in my backpack. Sometimes I bring along some nondairy milk, a bowl and spoon and enjoy the granola as cereal right on the trail! On its own or with milk, it's really satisfying and keeps you full a long time. The coconut extract (available online or at specialty spice shops) is optional, but since I discovered it, "optional" has become "mandatory" for me. Try this tasty addition in pancakes, soups, curries and more.

PREP TIME: 20 minutes
TOTAL TIME: 50 minutes
MAKES: 7 cups

EQUIPMENT
Large mixing bowl
Baking sheet lined with parchment paper
Small saucepan

INGREDIENTS
3 C. old-fashioned oats
½ C. all-purpose flour
1 TBS. brown sugar
1 TBS. ground flaxseed
(also called flaxseed meal)
1 TBS. hemp hearts
½ tsp. salt
1 tsp. cinnamon
½ C. pecans, chopped

½ C. slivered almonds
¼ C. sunflower seeds (raw or roasted/salted)
¼ C. pepitas (raw or roasted/salted)
½ cup unsweetened shredded coconut
½ C. nondairy butter
½ C. maple syrup
1 TBS. coconut oil
1 tsp. vanilla extract
1 tsp. natural coconut extract (optional)

DIRECTIONS
Preheat oven to 325°. In the large bowl, add the oats, flour, brown sugar, flaxseed, hemp hearts, salt and cinnamon and stir. Add the pecans, almonds, sunflower and pepitas, shredded coconut and stir. In the small saucepan on low heat add the butter, syrup, coconut oil and vanilla and coconut extracts. Stir and when completely melted, add to the mixture in the large mixing bowl and stir until coated evenly. Place the mixture on the baking sheet and spread out evenly. Bake for 20 minutes. Take out of the oven for a quick stir. Put back in the oven for 10 additional minutes or until golden brown. Allow plenty of time to cool. Store in an airtight container. This also freezes well for up to a month (if there's any left!).

GARDEN TRAIL MUFFINS

These savory muffins are made with fresh vegetables and a little kick of spice. They are light and fluffy yet really satisfying – either on their own or paired with a soup or salad. Make an easy meal for the trail by adding some fruit and nuts. Garden Trail Muffins are a great way to get vegetables in for those who are picky eaters! For your hike, place in an airtight container that will keep them from getting squashed.

PREP TIME: 30 minutes
TOTAL TIME: 55 minutes
MAKES: 12 standard sized muffins

EQUIPMENT
Muffin tin (12 muffins)
Large mixing bowl
2 small mixing bowls

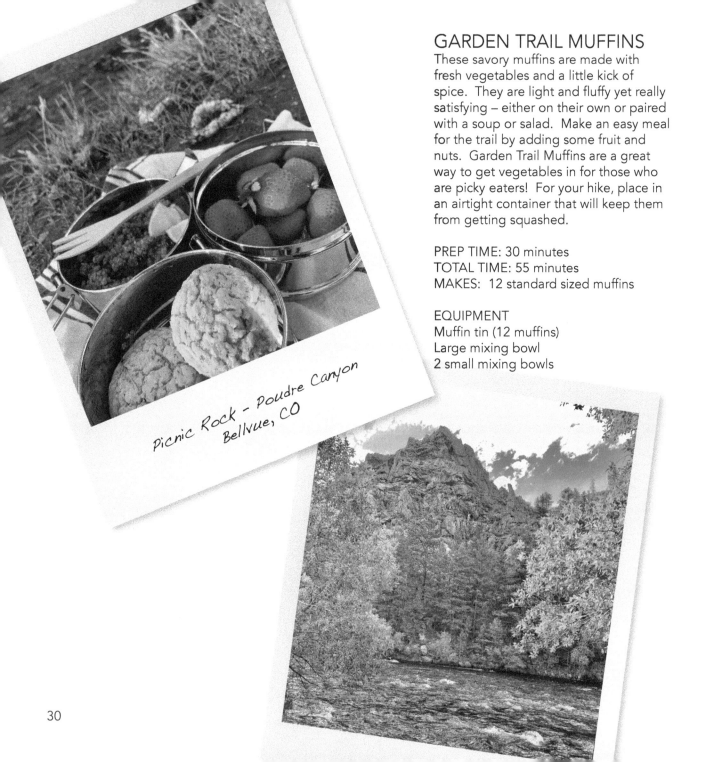

Picnic Rock – Poudre Canyon
Bellvue, CO

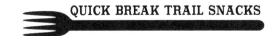

INGREDIENTS
Spray oil
1 C. all-purpose flour
1 C. garbanzo flour
1 TBS. nutritional yeast
1 1/2 tsp. baking powder
1/2 tsp. baking soda
Spice blend (recipe below)

1 C. nondairy milk
2 TBS. olive oil
Egg replacer (recipe below)
1 C. shredded zucchini (press with a towel to soak up excess water)
1 C. shredded carrots (press with a towel to soak up excess water)

EGG REPLACER
1 TBS. ground flaxseed (also called flaxseed meal)
3 TBS. water
Put ingredients in the small bowl, stir and set aside.

SPICE BLEND
2 tsp. salt
½ tsp. pepper
½ tsp. red pepper flakes (optional)
Combine all spice blend ingredients in the small bowl, stir and set aside.

DIRECTIONS
Preheat oven to 350°. Grease the muffin cup pans with the spray oil and set aside. In the large bowl add both of the flours, nutritional yeast, baking powder, baking soda and spice blend and stir. Add the milk, olive oil, egg replacer and stir. The batter consistency should be slightly thicker than pancake batter. Add the zucchini and carrots and stir. Spoon the batter into the muffin tins until about halfway filled. If there is additional batter, keep adding it evenly to the muffin tins so they all have about the same amount of batter. Top each muffin with a sprinkle of salt. Place in the oven for 25 minutes (test with a skewer to make sure the batter has fully cooked). Cool a few minutes then pop the muffins out of the muffin tin. Enjoy right away or after they are completely cooled, place in an airtight container until ready to use. These are best within two days, but you also have the option to freeze them.

TIP: when finished baking or after reheating, while they are still warm, cut in half and spread on a little nondairy butter or olive oil.

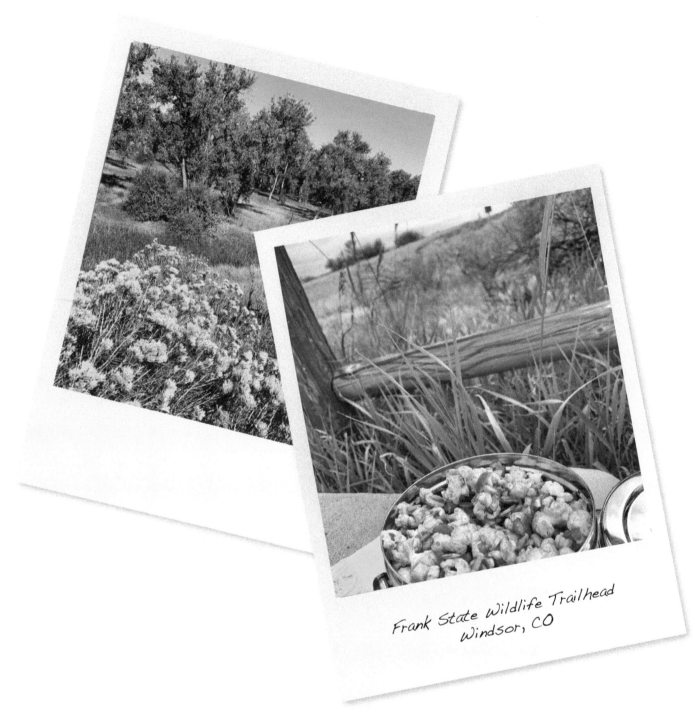

Frank State Wildlife Trailhead
Windsor, CO

TRAIL MIX POPCORN

There's so much crunchy and flavorful goodness in this popcorn! It's great for a snack or movie night at home or to bring out with you in nature. Place the cooled popcorn in an airtight container and take it along on your hike to enjoy. Bring a wet washcloth in case your hands get sticky!

PREP TIME: 30 minutes
TOTAL TIME: 40 minutes
MAKES: 7-8 cups

EQUIPMENT
Large, deep skillet with lid
Medium saucepan
Baking sheet lined with parchment paper

INGREDIENTS

⅓ C. popcorn kernels
1 TBS. coconut oil
¼ C. nondairy butter
¼ C. maple syrup
¼ C. brown sugar
3 TBS. almond butter
(or any nut butter variety)

1 tsp. vanilla
¼ tsp. cinnamon
¼ C. pepitas (raw or roasted)
¼ C. sunflower seeds (raw or roasted)
¼ C. slivered almonds
1 TBS. hemp hearts
½ tsp. salt

DIRECTIONS

Preheat oven to 300°. Heat oil in the skillet on medium/medium high heat. Put 2-3 kernels in the covered pan and wait for them to pop. When they pop take them out and put the rest of the kernels in the skillet. Shake the pan every so often so that the kernels don't burn. Leave the fully popped kernels in the skillet, turn off heat/remove from heat source and set aside. If you see any unpopped kernels, be sure to remove them. In the saucepan add the butter, maple syrup, brown sugar, almond butter, vanilla and cinnamon and stir on low heat until melted. Turn off the heat/remove from heat source. Add the pepitas, sunflower seeds, slivered almonds, hemp hearts and salt and stir. Pour mixture over the popcorn kernels in the skillet and gently fold with a rubber spatula. Put the popcorn mixture onto the baking sheet and place in the oven. Cook for 5 minutes, then turn the pan. Cook for another 5 minutes. Remove from the oven and allow to cool – leave plenty of time for this step so the popcorn hardens and is dry and crisp. Enjoy right away or put in an airtight container to enjoy within 3 days.

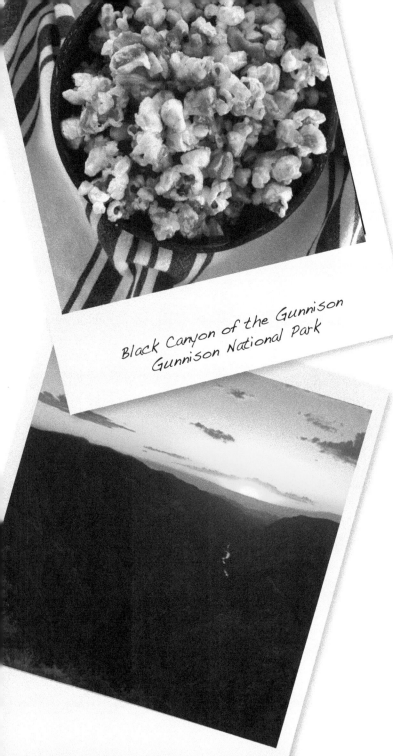

Black Canyon of the Gunnison
Gunnison National Park

HIGH WEST POPCORN

This addictive snack is named after the High West Saloon in Park City, Utah, which is known for its rustic-yet-luxurious style and décor, large selection of spirits and saloon-style fare. Not surprisingly, cashew and bacon popcorn is a popular starter on their menu. This vegan version is a gracious nod to the original, and without meat or dairy. Make sure it's stored in an airtight container, whether you keep it in your kitchen or bring it on the trail. Sticky hands on the trail may require a damp wash-cloth be added to your backpack.

PREP TIME: 50 minutes
TOTAL TIME: 1 hour
MAKES: 7-8 Cups

MAKE AHEAD: The coconut bacon and toasted cashews are great to make ahead. Store in an airtight container until ready to use.

EQUIPMENT
Large, deep skillet with lid
Medium saucepan
3 baking sheets lined with parchment paper
Rubber spatula

INGREDIENTS
1 C. toasted raw cashews (recipe below)
Coconut bacon (recipe, next page)
Skillet popcorn (recipe, next page)
Caramel sauce (recipe, next page)

TOASTED CASHEWS
Place nuts on the baking sheet and bake for 5 minutes or until golden brown and fragrant. They may need another minute or two of cooking time. Keep a close eye as they can burn easily. Allow to cool, then chop the cashews in large pieces and set aside.

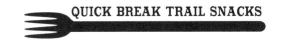

COCONUT BACON
Makes 2 cups (You'll use only ½ C. for the recipe – save the rest to enjoy later! It's wonderful to top off soup, avocado toast, dips, etc.)
2 TBS. liquid aminos (or soy sauce, or tamari)
½ TBS. maple syrup
½ tsp. smoked paprika
½ tsp. liquid smoke (optional)
¼ tsp. cayenne pepper
¼ tsp. salt
2 C. unsweetened flaked coconut
Preheat oven to 325°. In the mixing bowl add the aminos, maple syrup, paprika, liquid smoke, cayenne pepper and salt and stir. Fold in the coconut then pour mixture on the baking sheet. Bake for about 15 minutes, stirring every five minutes. Watch carefully to avoid burning. Allow to cool, then set aside.

POPCORN
⅓ C. popcorn kernels
1 TBS. coconut oil
Heat oil in the skillet on medium/medium high heat. To test the oil readiness, put 2 or 3 kernels in the covered pan and wait for them to pop. When they pop take them out and put the rest of the kernels in the skillet. Shake the pan every so often so that the kernels don't burn. Leave the fully popped kernels in the skillet, turn off heat/remove from heat source and set aside. If you see any unpopped kernels, be sure to remove them. Leave the popcorn in the skillet until the caramel sauce is ready.

CARAMEL SAUCE
¼ C. nondairy butter
2 TBS. C. maple syrup
½ C. brown sugar
1 tsp. vanilla
¼ tsp. cayenne pepper
½ tsp. salt
In the saucepan over low heat, add the butter, maple syrup, brown sugar, vanilla, cayenne pepper and salt. Stir until melted, then turn off the heat.

DIRECTIONS
Preheat oven to 300°. Add the toasted cashews and ½ C. coconut bacon to the caramel sauce and stir together. Pour mixture over the popcorn in the skillet and gently fold with a rubber spatula. Transfer the popcorn mixture to the baking sheet. Cook for 10 minutes, rotating the pan halfway through. Remove from the oven and set aside to cool – leave plenty of time for this step so that the popcorn hardens and is dry and crisp. Enjoy right away or put in an airtight container to enjoy within 3 days.

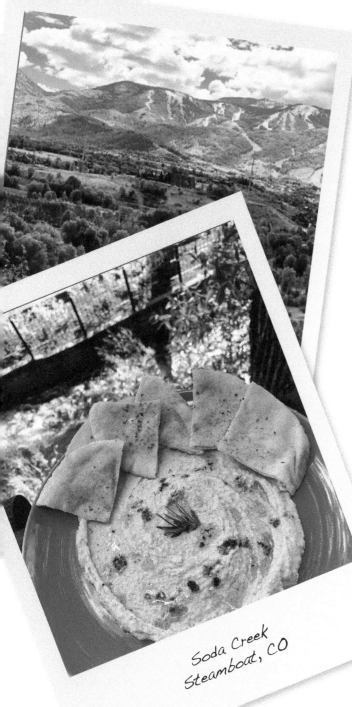

Soda Creek
Steamboat, CO

WHITE BEAN DIP
WITH ROASTED GARLIC AND RED CHILI OIL

The roasted garlic and red chili oil add smoky depth of flavor to this tasty, creamy dip. Serve it with toasted flatbread, tortilla chips or crackers – what a great pit-stop snack on the trail! The dip is also delicious spread on a bagel, in a veggie wrap or used as a base for avocado toast. Homemade flatbread is wonderful (p. 53) but if you are short on time, this recipe includes how to make the flatbread triangles with ready-made flatbread from your local market.

PREP TIME: 1 hour
TOTAL TIME: 1 hour 30 minutes
MAKES: 2 cups

MAKE AHEAD: The red chili oil, toasted cumin seeds and roasted garlic can all be made ahead to help save on time.

EQUIPMENT
Baking sheet lined with parchment paper
Food processor
Small frying pan
Aluminum foil
Mortar and pestle
Small saucepan
Small mixing bowl
Basting brush
Cutting board
Chef's knife
Pizza cutter

INGREDIENTS
1 can of cannellini beans, drained and rinsed
Roasted garlic (see recipe)
2 TBS. tahini
¼ C. olive oil
½ of a fresh squeezed lemon
2 tsp. toasted cumin seeds (see recipe, next page)
OR use ground cumin
½ tsp. salt
Red chili oil (see recipe, next page)
Flatbread triangles (see recipe, next page)

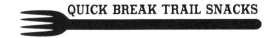

TOASTED CUMIN SEEDS
In the small frying pan, add the cumin seeds. Turn the heat on to medium and toast for 1-2 minutes, watching carefully so they don't burn. Turn off the heat and cool. Transfer the seeds to a mortar and pestle and grind to a fine powder.

ROASTED GARLIC
Whole head of garlic
Olive oil
Preheat oven to 350°. Place the head of garlic on a cutting board and trim the top of the cloves about ½". Place on a small sheet of foil, drizzle with olive oil, wrap it up in the foil and seal the edges. Cook for 30 minutes. Remove from the oven and cool completely. If making this ahead, store in the refrigerator until use, up to 2-3 days.

RED CHILI OIL
½ C. olive oil
1 tsp. red pepper flakes
Pinch of salt
Add the oil, pepper flakes and salt to the saucepan. Heat on low for 10 minutes, then turn off heat/remove from heat source to cool. The pepper flakes can remain in the oil or you can strain them. Put in an airtight container and store in the refrigerator for up to 3-4 weeks.

FLATBREAD TRIANGLES
1 package of flatbread from the grocery store (or make your own, see recipe P. 53)
2 TBS. olive oil
Pinch of salt
Pinch of dried oregano
Preheat oven to 400°. In the small mixing bowl, add the olive oil, salt and oregano and stir. Place the flatbread pieces on a baking sheet without overlapping too much. Use the basting brush to brush each flatbread with the olive oil mixture. Bake for 10 minutes, or until they are thoroughly warmed. Allow to cool slightly, then cut into triangle shaped pieces with the pizza cutter or sharp knife. Serve right away or store for later. If storing, cool completely then place in an airtight container wherever you store bread for up to 2-3 days.

DIRECTIONS
Put the beans, roasted garlic (squeeze from the bottom of the bulb to remove the garlic cloves from the skin/outer layers), tahini, olive oil, lemon juice, cumin and salt in the food processor. Blend until creamy and smooth. Taste, and add salt if needed. After plating, drizzle with the red chili oil – the more you add, the spicier it gets! If packing it up for the trail, add the red chili oil beforehand so it's ready for dipping.

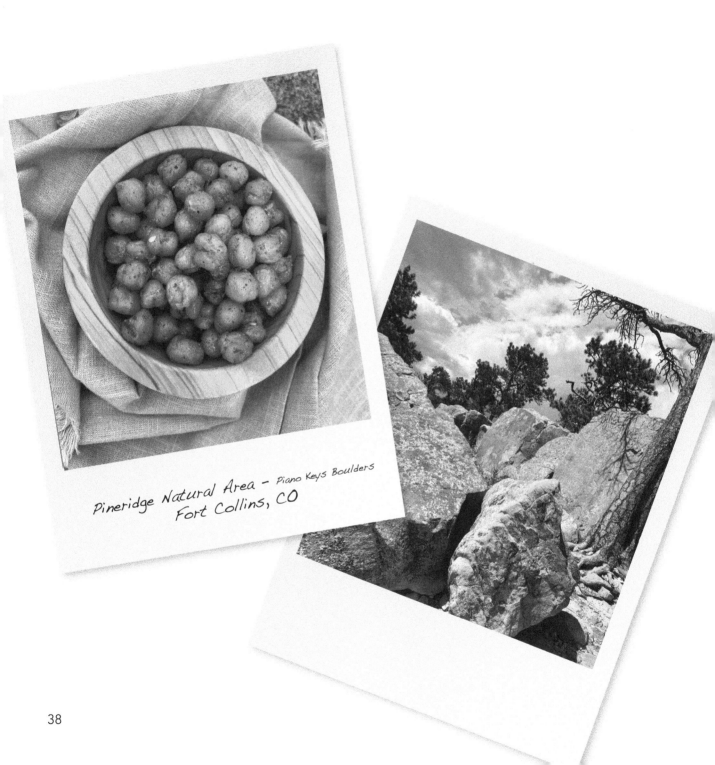

Pineridge Natural Area – Piano Keys Boulders
Fort Collins, CO

38

CRISPY CHICKPEAS

These crispy little bites are so yummy to take on a hike. But here's a warning: You'll want to eat them all when they're fresh out of the oven, but you can't or you won't have any for the trail! After they are cooled, they can be stored in an airtight container. The chickpeas are not as crispy if not eaten right away, but they are still flavorful and delicious. Great to top off a soup or salad, too! This is also a fun opportunity to experiment with creating your own custom spice blend.

PREP TIME: 20 minutes
TOTAL TIME: 1 hour
MAKES: 2 cups

EQUIPMENT
Large mixing bowl
Small mixing bowl
Colander
1 clean kitchen towel
Baking sheet lined with parchment paper

INGREDIENTS
2 cans of chickpeas, rinsed and drained Lay them out on a clean kitchen towel and gently massage them to encourage the skins to be removed. This step will make the chickpeas crispier! Don't worry about getting them all, just try for most.)
¼ C. avocado oil
Spice blend (suggested recipe below)

SPICE BLEND
1 TBS. za'tar (OR 1 tsp. sesame seeds, 1 tsp. cumin, 1 tsp. chili powder, ½ tsp. salt,
½ tsp. garlic powder)
1 tsp. salt
¼ tsp. ground black pepper
Combine all spice blend ingredients in the small bowl, stir and set aside.

DIRECTIONS
Preheat oven to 375°. In the large bowl mix together the oil and spice blend. Add the chickpeas and gently stir so they are all well coated. Place chickpeas on the baking sheet and cook in the oven for 40 minutes, giving the pan a little shake every 15 minutes. Keep a close eye on them during the last 10 minutes so they don't overcook. They may be ready sooner than the full cooking time.

GREEN LENTIL HUMMUS

If you've just had hummus only made from chickpeas, you're in for a big treat! Got time to make homemade flatbread for dipping? Trust me, it's worth it! Head to the recipe on P.53. Otherwise, grab some flatbread at the grocery store – or crackers or tortilla chips – and chow down. Try the hummus in a wrap with fresh vegetables for a handheld meal on the trail.

PREP TIME: 30 minutes
TOTAL TIME: 1 hour
MAKES: 3 ½ cups

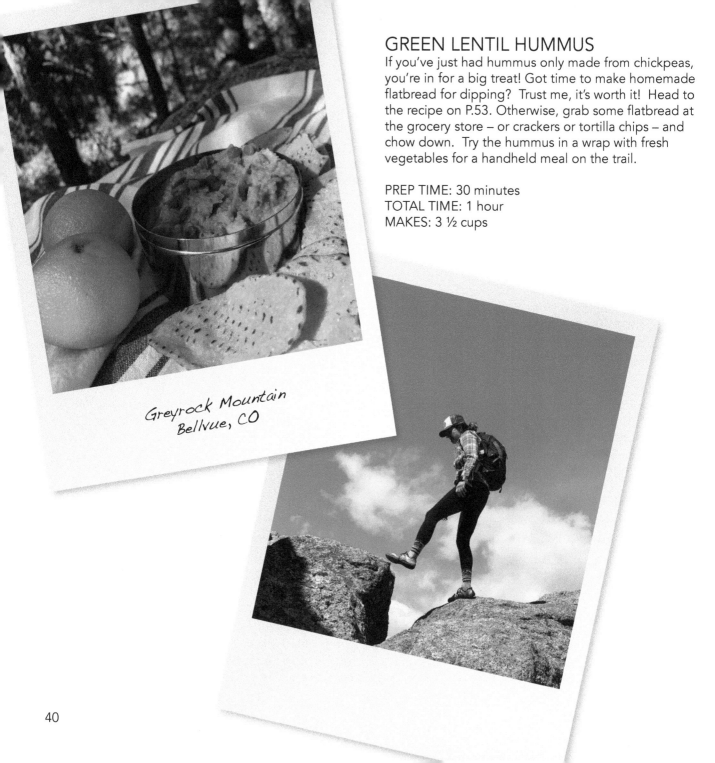

Greyrock Mountain
Bellvue, CO

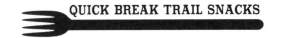

EQUIPMENT
Colander
Kitchen towel
2 small mixing bowls
Medium saucepan with lid
Small frying pan
Large bowl
Mortar and pestle (optional)
Food processor (a blender can also work)

INGREDIENTS
1 can of chickpeas, rinsed and drained. Lay them out on a clean kitchen towel and gently massage them to encourage the skins to come off. This step will make the hummus creamier!
½ C. green lentils, rinsed
1 ½ C. water
2 tsp. cumin seeds
¼ C. olive oil + more as needed
Spice blend (recipe below)
2 cloves fresh garlic, minced
½ of a fresh lime, squeezed

SPICE BLEND
2 tsp. freshly ground toasted cumin seeds (or pre-ground)
¼ tsp. red pepper flakes (optional)
¼ tsp. turmeric
½ tsp. salt
Heat the frying pan on medium. Add the cumin seeds and toast until fragrant, about 1-2 minutes. Turn off the heat/remove from heat source and cool. When cooled, place in the mortar and pestle and grind until powdery. Combine all spice blend ingredients in the small bowl, stir and set aside.

DIRECTIONS
In the saucepan, add the green lentils and water. Bring to a boil then cover and simmer for 20-25 minutes. Check them to make sure they are soft/al dente, then drain and set aside. In the other small bowl, reserve 3 tablespoons of the lentils and set aside. In the food processor, add the chickpeas and the cooked green lentils (remember to keep the reserved lentils aside), olive oil, spice blend, garlic and lime juice and blend on high until very creamy. You may need to add a little more olive oil to get the consistency you desire. Place the hummus in the large mixing bowl and gently fold in the reserved lentils. Take a taste to see if you need to adjust the seasonings. Top with a sprinkle of salt and drizzle of olive oil.

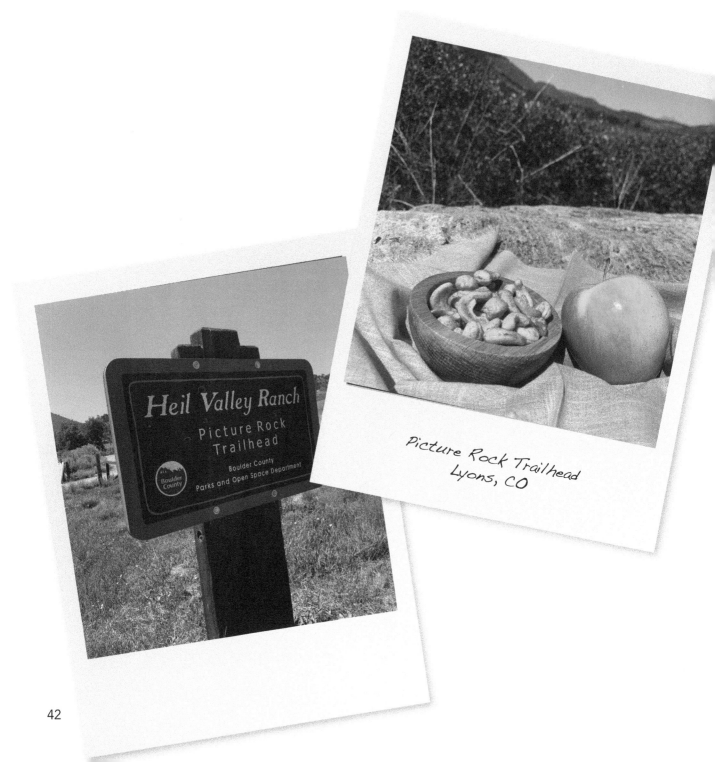

Picture Rock Trailhead
Lyons, CO

Heil Valley Ranch
Picture Rock
Trailhead

Boulder County
Parks and Open Space Department

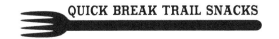

INDIAN-SPICED CASHEWS

These good-for-you baked nuts are so tempting, and are perfect in salads, wraps, as a topping on soup or on their own as a snack. So versatile! Customize this recipe to suit your palette by dialing down or turning up the heat using more or less chili and curry powder. Nuts and a piece of fruit make a great pair on the trail!

PREP TIME: 15 minutes
TOTAL TIME: 25 minutes
MAKES: 2 cups

EQUIPMENT
Medium mixing bowl
Baking sheet lined with parchment paper
Small mixing bowl

INGREDIENTS
2 C. raw cashews
1 ½ TBS. olive oil
Spice blend (see recipe below)

SPICE BLEND
1 heaping tsp. curry powder
½ tsp. ground cumin
¼ tsp. turmeric
Up to ¼ tsp. Indian chili powder (This very hot spice is easily found online or at Indian markets. Use cayenne pepper as a substitute.)
½ tsp. salt, plus more if needed
Combine all spice blend ingredients in the small bowl, stir and set aside.

DIRECTIONS
Preheat oven to 350°. In the medium bowl, add nuts and oil. Stir until lightly coated. Add the spice blend and stir until the nuts are well coated. Arrange the nuts on the baking sheet evenly so they don't overlap. Place in the oven for 5-7 minutes keeping a close eye so they don't burn. Enjoy the lovely aroma that fills your kitchen! Allow the nuts to cool completely before eating or storing in an airtight container.

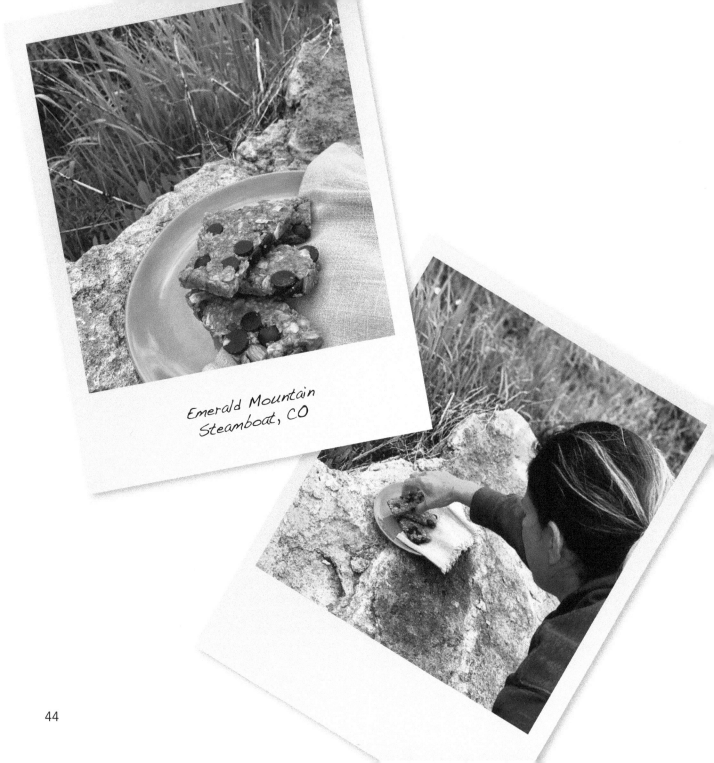

Emerald Mountain
Steamboat, CO

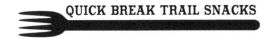

ALMOND BLISS BARS

These no-bake bars are fast and easy to make – perfect to pop out of the freezer and hit the trail, or for a quick snack at home. The almonds, coconut and chocolate are reminiscent of the treasured candy bar, but this version is made with healthier ingredients. My teenage boys are fans and request them frequently.

PREP TIME: 30 minutes
TOTAL TIME: 1 hour, 30 minutes
MAKES: 24 bars (1.75" length, 3.5" width, just over 1/4" thick)

EQUIPMENT
9 x 12" baking pan, lined with parchment paper (so that there are a few inches of extra paper hanging over the sides of the pan)
Food processor
Large mixing bowl
Cutting board
Chef's knife

INGREDIENTS
2 C. old-fashioned rolled oats, divided
2 TBS. coconut flour (or use all-purpose flour as a substitute)
2 TBS. hemp hearts
2 TBS. ground flaxseed (also called flaxseed meal)
½ C. pure maple syrup
1 C. unsweetened shredded coconut
1 C. dry roasted almonds, chopped
1 tsp. vanilla
1 C. almond butter
1 C. nondairy dark chocolate chips

DIRECTIONS
In the food processor, add 1 cup of the rolled oats and blend on high until powdery (the pulsated oats turn into oat flour). In the large mixing bowl, stir together the oat flour, rolled oats, coconut flour, hemp hearts, ground flaxseed, maple syrup, coconut, almonds, vanilla, almond butter and chocolate chips. Empty the mixture into the pan. Press down with your hands so that all the mixture is mostly an even thickness. Cover and place in the freezer for an hour or longer. Remove the bars from the pan (by holding on to the parchment paper overhang) and place on a cutting board. Cut the bars to your desired size. Store in a container in the refrigerator for up to 3 days, or tightly wrapped in the freezer for up to a month.

BUDDHA BURGERS WITH SPICY AIOLI

This hearty dish will fill your tank on the trail – a perfect meal to refuel during a demanding hike, or to celebrate your accomplishment at the end. Bring along extra napkins and perhaps some utensils – the dish can get messy, but it's worth it! Buns and toppings should be packed separately; assemble the burgers when ready to eat. Sweet Potato Slices with Sweet Mustard Sauce recipe follows this one, the perfect companion to the Buddha Burger! Take a moment to read through the whole recipe before getting started.

PREP TIME: 45 minutes
TOTAL: 1 hour, 15 minutes
MAKES: 6 burger patties

MAKE AHEAD: Chop the vegetables and/or make the aioli the day before and refrigerate (up to 3 days) until ready to use.

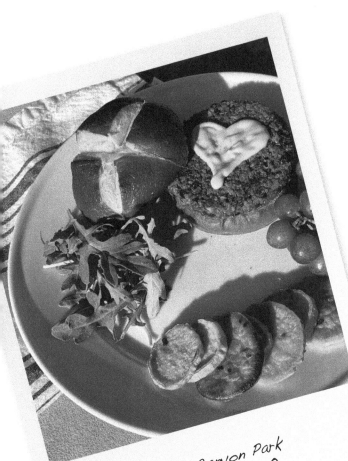

Spring Canyon Park
Fort Collins, CO

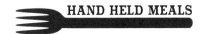

EQUIPMENT
Medium saucepan with lid
Large skillet
Cutting board
Chef's knife
Large mixing bowl
Medium mixing bowl
3 small mixing bowls
Potato masher (or large fork)

INGREDIENTS
3 TBS. olive oil, divided
½ C. onion, diced
2 garlic cloves, minced
1 jalapeño pepper (optional), with or without seeds, diced
1 C. broccoli, chopped
1 C. carrots, chopped
1 C. bell pepper, chopped
1 can black beans, drained and rinsed
1 C. cooked quinoa (recipe below)
Egg replacer (recipe below)
¼ C. raw sunflower seeds
Spice blend (recipe below)
Optional serving suggestions, see next page

QUINOA
½ C. dry quinoa
1 C. vegetable broth
In the medium saucepan, add quinoa and water. Bring to a boil then reduce heat and simmer, covered, for 15 minutes. Turn off heat/remove from heat source, leave covered, and let stand for 10 minutes.

EGG REPLACER
1 TBS. ground flaxseed (also called flaxseed meal)
3 TBS. water
Put ingredients in the small bowl, stir and set aside.

(continued, next page)

SPICE BLEND
1 tsp. cumin
1 tsp. chili powder
1 tsp. salt
Combine all spice blend ingredients in the small bowl, stir and set aside.

DIRECTIONS
Heat the skillet on medium heat. Add 2 TBS. olive oil. When the oil is heated, add the onion and cook until soft, 2-3 minutes. Add the garlic and jalapeño and stir; cook for 1 minute. Add the broccoli, carrots and bell pepper and cook for 2-3 more minutes, or until soft. Turn off the heat and transfer the vegetable mixture to the large mixing bowl. In the medium mixing bowl, add the black beans and mash them with a potato masher or large fork until there is a coarse consistency (leave some of the black beans whole). Add the black beans, ground flax seed mixture, spice blend, sunflower seeds and quinoa to the vegetable mixture in the large mixing bowl and stir. Taste and add more salt if needed. On medium, heat the same skillet (no need to wash it) and add the remaining 1 TBS. oil. While the oil is heating, form ½ C. of the burger mixture into patties with your hands. Add the patties to the skillet and cook until golden brown on each side. Cook in two batches if all the burgers don't fit in your skillet with space between.

PLATING
place the patties on toasted buns (if using), along with the sweet potatoes and your choice of toppings.

SPICY AIOLI
¼ C. nondairy mayonnaise
½ tsp. (or more, to your liking) hot sauce
Mix the mayo and the hot sauce in the small mixing bowl and stir until completely blended.

SERVING IDEAS TOPPINGS
Burger buns, toasted
Mixed greens
Sliced tomato
Sliced avocado
Nondairy mayo
Nondairy cheese
Pickles

SWEET POTATO SLICES WITH SWEET MUSTARD SAUCE

These are awesome straight from the pan or to bring along on a hike served up with the sweet mustard sauce. The spiciness of the mustard sauce compliments the sweet potatoes, especially if you choose to use the red pepper flakes.

PREP TIME: 15 minutes
TOTAL: 45 minutes
SERVES: 6

MAKE AHEAD: Prepare the sweet mustard sauce and store in the refrigerator until ready to use.

EQUIPMENT
Baking sheet lined with parchment paper
Medium bowl
Whisk
Cutting board
Chef's knife

INGREDIENTS
1 large sweet potato, cut into ½" thick slices (skin on or peeled)
Avocado oil
Red pepper flakes (optional)
Salt to taste
Sweet Mustard Sauce (recipe below)

SWEET MUSTARD SAUCE
½ C. nondairy mayo
2 TBS. agave nectar or other sweetener
1 TBS. Dijon mustard
½ TBS. white vinegar or lemon juice
In the medium bowl, add all the ingredients and whisk until blended. Store in the refrigerator for up to 3 days.

DIRECTIONS
Preheat oven to 400°. Place the sweet potato slices ½" apart on the baking sheet. On both sides, drizzle with oil then sprinkle with red pepper flakes and salt. Bake for 35 minutes or until the edges are browned and the center is fork-tender.

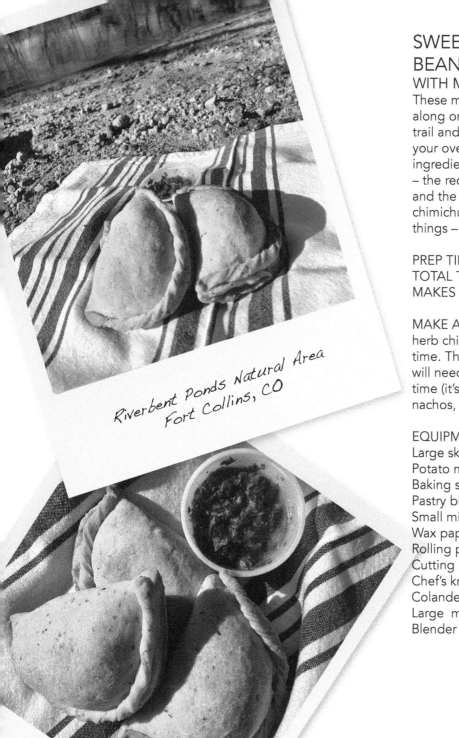

Riverbent Ponds Natural Area
Fort Collins, CO

SWEET POTATO AND BLACK BEAN EMPANADAS
WITH MIXED-HERB CHIMICHURRI

These meals-in-a-pocket are perfect for toting along on your hike. They're great cold on the trail and will also reheat wonderfully later in your oven. Don't be thrown by the number of ingredients and process of making the dough – the recipe is nearly impossible to mess up, and the results are beyond delicious! The chimichurri is a great condiment on so many things – try it on a protein or with pasta.

PREP TIME: 1 hours
TOTAL TIME: 2 hours
MAKES 12 empanadas

MAKE AHEAD: The filling and the mixed herb chimichurri can be made a day ahead of time. The recipe makes more filling than you will need. You can freeze the rest for another time (it's perfect for use in enchiladas, tacos, nachos, etc.)

EQUIPMENT
Large skillet
Potato masher (optional)
Baking sheet lined with parchment paper
Pastry blender (or a fork)
Small mixing bowl
Wax paper
Rolling pin
Cutting board
Chef's knife
Colander
Large mixing bowl
Blender

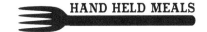

INGREDIENTS
Empanada dough (recipe below)
Mixed Herb Chimichurri
Empanada filling (recipe, next page)

EMPANADA DOUGH
TIP: Make the dough first, and while it's chilling in the fridge, make the empanada filling.

2 ¼ C. all-purpose flour (plus extra for rolling out the dough)
1 tsp. baking powder
1 ½ tsp. salt
1 stick of very cold nondairy butter
⅓ C. ice water
1 TBS. white vinegar
1 egg replacer (recipe below)
Spray oil

EGG REPLACER
1 TBS. ground flaxseed (also called flaxseed meal)
3 TBS. water
Put ingredients in the small bowl, stir and set aside.

DIRECTIONS
In the large mixing bowl, stir together the flour, baking powder and salt. Add the butter and with a pastry blender, blend until coarsely crumbled. Add the ice water and vinegar to the flour mix, and the egg replacer. Mix until the dough starts to come together. On a clean and lightly-floured surface, knead the dough a few times. Form into a large ball. Wrap in wax paper and place in the fridge. Clean up your space and begin to make the empanada filling while the dough is chilling.

MIXED HERB CHIMICHURRI
2 C of mixed fresh herbs such as flat leaf parsley, cilantro, oregano, basil
¼ C. olive oil, plus more as needed
2 garlic cloves
1 TBS. fresh lemon juice
½ tsp. red pepper flakes
½ tsp. salt
Pulse in a blender until well combined. Place in an airtight container and place in the fridge. Use within three days, or freeze for up to one month.

(continued, next page)

EMPANADA FILLING
2 TBS. olive oil
½ onion, diced
1 jalapeño pepper (optional), with or without seeds, diced
4 cloves garlic, minced
1 medium sweet potato, peeled and cubed
2 large yellow potatoes, peeled and cubed
1 tsp. salt
1 tsp. cumin
¼ C. water
1 can of black beans, rinsed and drained
¼ C. olive oil

DIRECTIONS
In a large skillet on medium heat, add the olive oil. When the skillet is hot, add the onion and stir. Cook for 2-3 minutes. Add the jalapeño and garlic and stir. Cook for an additional 1-2 minutes. Add the sweet and yellow potatoes, salt, cumin and water. Stir and cover. Cook on medium heat for 15 minutes or until they soften. Add the black beans, stir and cook for 1-2 minutes. When finished cooking, turn off the heat/remove from heat source. Mash down about ½ of the mixture with a potato masher or fork. Add the olive oil and stir. Taste and add more salt if needed. Set aside.

Preheat oven to 400°. Take the dough out of the fridge, unwrap it then put it on a clean and floured surface. Dust the dough ball with flour, then roll until very thin, about $\frac{1}{16}$". Use a large glass jar or a small bowl (about 5" in diameter) to cut out the circles. You should have a bit of left over dough to create the fancy edging if you like – just use a small strip of dough and twirl it around and place on the edge of the filled empanada. Not mandatory, but fun to do and looks pretty. Depending on the size of your dough circles, you will need to adjust the amount of filling (I created 5" dough circles and put 1 ½ TBS. of filling in each one). Seal the edges with your fingertips. Add the "fancy" edge with the extra dough (or skip it). You can also press the edges with a fork to create lines. Place each filled empanada on the baking sheet.

Spray the finished empanadas lightly with the oil and place in oven for 15 minutes or until golden brown. You may need additional cooking time; just be careful to keep a close eye so they don't start to burn. Cool and serve with the chimichurri, or store in the fridge. These freeze well for later.

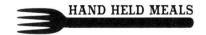

HOMEMADE FLATBREAD

PREP TIME: 3 hours
TOTAL TIME: 3 hours and 30 minutes
MAKES: 8 pieces of homemade flatbread

EQUIPMENT
Countertop mixer with dough hook attachment,
whisk attachment
Spatula
Rolling pin
Cast iron skillet
Large mixing bowl
Whisk

INGREDIENTS
½ TBS. sugar
1 package of active dry yeast (equivalent to 2 ¼ tsp.)
1 C. lukewarm water
3 C. all-purpose flour, divided, plus extra for dusting
the rolling surface
1 TBS. olive oil
1 ½ tsp. salt
Cooking spray

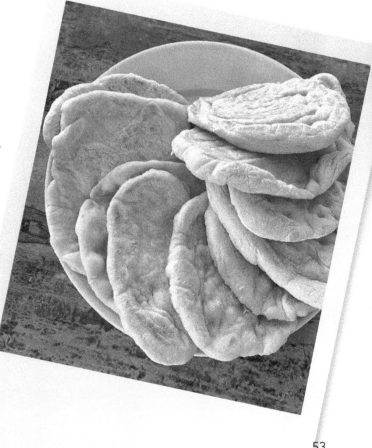

DIRECTIONS
In the countertop mixing bowl, add the sugar, yeast,
lukewarm water and 1 C. of the flour and manually
whisk or use the countertop mixer whisk attachment
until blended. Cover the bowl with a kitchen towel
and set aside for 15 minutes in a warm, dry area (the
mixture will be foamy). Add the olive oil, salt and
1 ½ C. flour. Turn the mixer on low speed and mix
until the dough forms – there is a reserve of ½ C.
flour in case any additional flour is needed. Keep
the mixer on low and allow for it to stir for about
5 minutes. Remove the dough, place on a floured
surface and form into the shape of a ball. Place the
dough ball in a lightly oiled large bowl and cover
with a kitchen towel. Set in a warm, dry area for 2
hours. The dough should double in size. Cut the
dough evenly into 8 pieces and form each piece
into a small ball. Roll each small ball with a rolling
pin until the dough is ¼" thick. Drizzle or spray oil
in a cast iron skillet over medium heat. Add the
flatbread dough and cook until it begins to puff up.
Just as it starts to brown, flip the bread and cook on
the other side until golden brown. Serve quickly or
allow to cool then store in an airtight container. It
will keep fresh for 2-3 days.

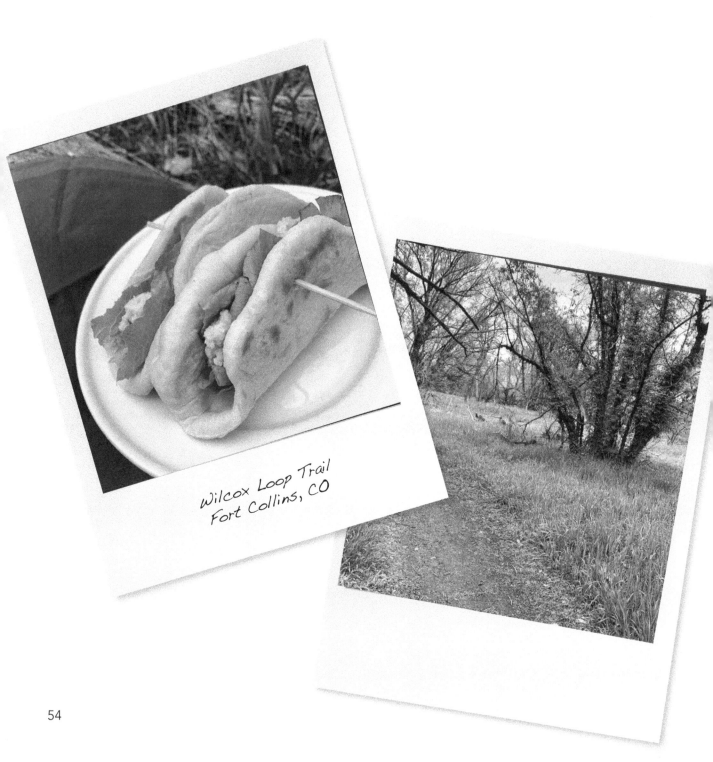

Wilcox Loop Trail
Fort Collins, CO

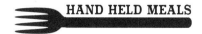

CHICKPEA CURRY SALAD ON FLATBREAD

This chickpea curry has a wonderful balance of curry and cilantro, and it's easy to wrap up and take on a hike for a satisfying break. The flatbread can be made at home (P. 53) or bought in the store. Our teenage boys devour the homemade version – you may need to hide it until you are ready to use! You can also serve the chickpea curry salad on sandwich bread or in a wrap. Additionally, it is a fantastic dip to bring to parties – serve with tortilla chips, crackers or the homemade flatbread cut into small triangles.

PREP TIME: 10 minutes
TOTAL TIME: 15 minutes
SERVES: 2

EQUIPMENT
Large fork or potato masher utensil
Medium mixing bowl
Small mixing bowl

INGREDIENTS
1 can of chickpeas, drained and rinsed
2 TBS. nondairy mayonnaise
½ C. cilantro, chopped
Spice blend (see below)
Fresh lime juice
Lettuce (any variety)

SPICE BLEND
½ tsp. curry powder
¼ tsp. salt
¼ tsp. cayenne pepper
Combine all spice blend ingredients in the small bowl, stir and set aside.

DIRECTIONS
Put the chickpeas into the medium bowl. Mash them using the back of a large fork or a potato masher so that most are mashed, but some are only partially mashed for texture. Add the mayo and spice blend and stir until mixed. Add the chopped cilantro and stir. Add a squeeze of fresh lime juice, stir, then taste and add salt if needed. Line the flatbread with a leaf of fresh lettuce. Add a scoop of the chickpea salad, then fold in half and enjoy.

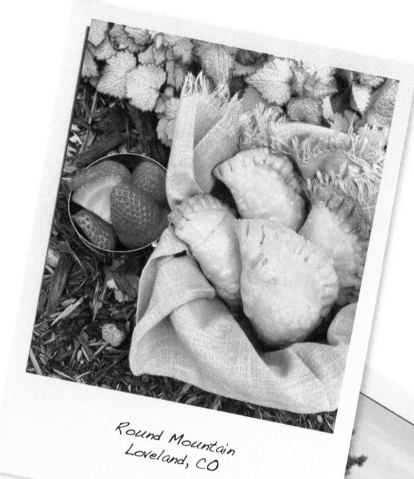

Round Mountain
Loveland, CO

SHEPHERD'S HAND PIES

A twist on traditional shepherd's pie, these hand-held pies are stuffed with healthy and protein-rich lentils instead of meat, plus mashed potatoes, vegetables and a kiss of rosemary. This recipe is made easy and quick by using canned lentils, store-bought piecrusts and frozen veggies. Right out of the oven or wrapped individually for the trail, these little pies will please and fill your belly.

PREP TIME: 45 minutes
TOTAL TIME: 1 hour, 10 minutes
MAKES: 22-24 4" pies

MAKE AHEAD: Prepare the filling and mashed potatoes a day ahead of time.

EQUIPMENT
Cutting board
Chef's knife
Medium saucepan
Colander
Potato masher or large fork
Large, deep skillet
Rolling pin
4" round biscuit cutter
Basting brush
Baking sheet lined with parchment paper

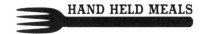

INGREDIENTS
1 box of frozen nondairy piecrusts (2 crusts/pkg) thawed to room temp (3-4 hours)
2 lbs. Yukon gold potatoes, peeled and quartered
2 tsp. salt, divided
1 stick (8 TBS.) of nondairy butter, divided
½ tsp. ground black pepper
1 TBS olive oil
½ medium onion, diced
2 cloves of garlic, minced
2 C. mushrooms, sliced
1 tsp. liquid aminos or soy sauce
10 oz. bag of frozen classic vegetables (cubed carrots, peas, corn) or chopped fresh vegetables
1 15 oz. can of brown lentils, drained and rinsed
1 C. vegetable broth
2 sprigs of fresh rosemary (4-5" long each)

DIRECTIONS
Preheat oven to 400°. In the medium saucepan, add the potatoes and 1 tsp. salt. Fill with cold water about 1" above the potatoes. Turn heat on high until boiling. Reduce heat to low then simmer, uncovered, for 20 minutes until done (you should be able to insert a fork easily into the potatoes). Drain in the colander. Place the drained potatoes back into the saucepan. Add 4 TBS. butter, 1 tsp. salt and the ground pepper. Mash with the potato masher or fork until blended and creamy. Set aside.

Heat the skillet to medium heat with the oil and 4 TBS. butter. Add the onion and cook for 2-3 minutes, or until soft. Add the garlic, mushrooms and aminos and cook for 2-3 minutes. Add the frozen vegetables, lentils, vegetable broth and stir. Add the rosemary sprigs and stir gently. Turn the heat down to low and simmer for 20 minutes (uncovered). Remove the rosemary sprigs and discard after cooking. Taste and add salt/pepper as needed.

While the vegetable/lentil mixture is cooking, unwrap the thawed piecrust dough. Roll out the dough to about ¹⁄₁₆". Cut into the dough with the biscuit cutter until all the piecrust dough is used up. Add 2 teaspoons of mashed potatoes and 2 teaspoons of vegetable/lentil filling. Fold the dough in half then press down with a fork to secure the edges. Arrange on the baking sheet and use the basting brush to brush water on the tops of the pies. Place in the oven for 15-20 minutes, until golden brown. Allow time to cool, then serve.

TIP: If the piecrust is holding you back, skip it! Preheat the oven to 400° and put the mixture in a greased 9 x 12" pan and top evenly with the mashed potatoes. Cook for 20 minutes, or until the top of the mashed potatoes starts to brown.

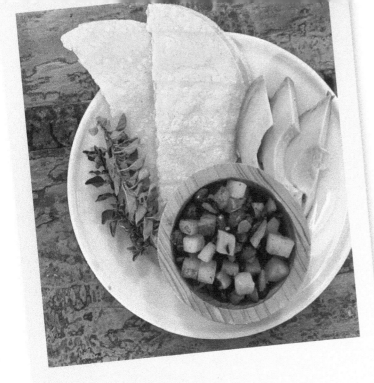

The Livingroom Trailhead
Salt Lake City, Utah

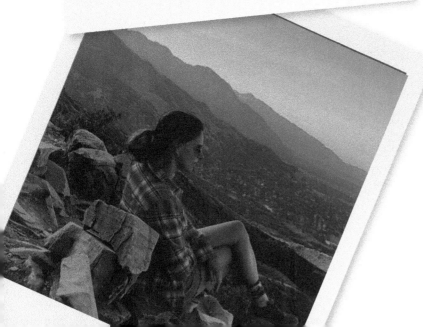

BREAKFAST (or lunch, or dinner)
POTATO HASH
WITH CREAMY TAHINI

I have been making this at any time of the day for years. This recipe offers wonderful memories of all the times I have taken this out with me in nature and how much the tahini sauce and fresh herbs have made this a favorite. The hash is easy to take along in a wrap, a big scoop in a salad, or as a side dish to compliment a main meal.

PREP TIME: 20 minutes
TOTAL TIME: 45 minutes
SERVES: 6

MAKE AHEAD: The creamy tahini sauce can be made ahead and stored in the refrigerator for up to 3 days. It's also wonderful for dipping vegetables or as a replacement for mayonnaise on a sandwich.

EQUIPMENT
Colander
Cutting board
Chef's knife
Small mixing bowl
Large skillet
Medium mixing bowl
Whisk

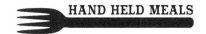

INGREDIENTS
2 TBS. olive oil
½ onion, diced
1 medium sweet potato, peeled and cubed
2 medium Yukon gold potatoes, peeled and cubed
1 can of pinto beans, rinsed and drained
Spice blend (see recipe below)
1 C. chopped herbs (such as cilantro, oregano or parsley)
Avocado slices
Leafy green lettuce (such as romaine, arugula, butterhead, spinach), rinsed and trimmed
Hot sauce (optional)
Flour or corn tortillas

SPICE BLEND
1 tsp. salt
1 tsp. ground cumin
¼ tsp. turmeric
½ tsp. garlic powder
½ tsp. cayenne pepper (optional)
Combine all spice blend ingredients in the small bowl, stir and set aside.

CREAMY TAHINI SAUCE
½ C. tahini
¼ C. water
¼ tsp. salt
¼ C. cilantro, chopped
In the medium mixing bowl, add the tahini, water and salt. Whisk until creamy and well blended. Add the cilantro and stir gently. Set aside, or refrigerate if not using right away.

DIRECTIONS
Heat oil on medium high in the skillet. Add the onion and cook for 2-3 minutes. Add the sweet and Yukon gold potatoes. Cook for 15 minutes (stirring occasionally), or until fork-tender (you may need some extra time). Add the spice blend and beans, then stir and cook for 2-3 minutes. Turn off heat/ remove from heat source. Add the chopped herbs and stir.

PLATING
With the tortilla open and flat on your plate, add the lettuce and a generous scoop of the hash. Top with avocado, hot sauce and the creamy tahini. Wrap it up and enjoy right away or roll it up in parchment paper or foil to enjoy later on the trail.

VEGETABLE VINDALOO FLATBREAD

In this flatbread sandwich, traditional flavors from India are paired with the coolness of yogurt sauce and nuttiness of tahini (ground sesame seeds). It's your choice to make the flatbread from scratch (see P. 53 for the recipe) or to buy some already made from the store. To assemble your flatbread for a hike, roll it up in parchment paper or foil and secure with a toothpick or bamboo skewer – a very tasty reward for your effort on the trail.

PREP: 40 minutes
TOTAL: 1 hour
MAKES: 3 servings

MAKE AHEAD: Prepare the spice blend, tzatziki and tahini sauces in advance for less time in the kitchen when you are ready to prepare your meal.

EQUIPMENT
Colander
Large skillet
3 small bowls
Large mixing bowl

INGREDIENTS
3 TBS. olive oil, divided
1 C. kale, rinsed, trimmed and chopped into very small, bite sized pieces
1 portabello mushroom, thinly sliced (or 2 C. sliced mushrooms of any variety)
1 C. red onion, thinly sliced
½ C. carrots, shredded
2 tsp. cumin seeds
1 tsp. mustard seeds
Spice Blend (recipe next page)
1 can of chickpeas, drained and rinsed
Tzatziki sauce (recipe next page)
Tahini sauce (recipe next page)
Flatbread bread (recipe on P. 53 or store bought)

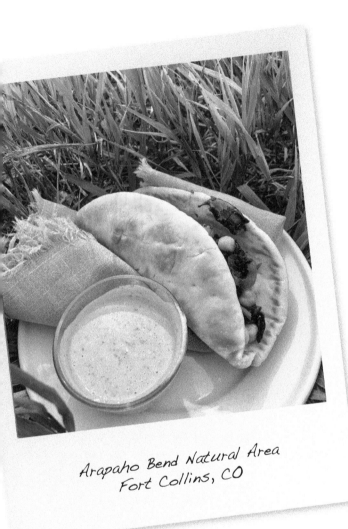

Arapaho Bend Natural Area
Fort Collins, CO

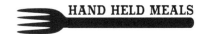

SPICE BLEND
1 tsp. salt
½ tsp. ground coriander
½ tsp. turmeric
¼ tsp. cumin
½ tsp. garlic powder
½ tsp. red chili powder or cayenne pepper
½ tsp. ground ginger
Small pinch of cinnamon
Combine all spice blend ingredients in the small bowl, stir and set aside. Reserve ½ tsp. of the spice blend for the tzatziki sauce.

TZATZIKI SAUCE
2 TBS. nondairy yogurt
½ tsp. reserved spice blend
1 tsp. olive oil
Add yogurt, reserved spice blend and olive oil to the small bowl. Cover and keep in the fridge until ready to use, can also be stored in the refrigerator a day in advance.

TAHINI SAUCE
½ C. tahini
1 tsp. salt
¼ C. water, plus additional for desired consistency)
Stir together tahini, salt and water in the small bowl. Cover and keep in the fridge until ready to use, can also be stored in the refrigerator a day in advance.

DIRECTIONS
In the large bowl add kale and 2 TBS. olive oil. With your hands, massage the kale so that the oil is evenly distributed and the kale begins to break down. Add the mushrooms, onion and carrots to the bowl, stir, set aside. Heat 1 TBS. olive oil in the skillet on medium. Add the cumin and mustard seeds. Cook for 1-2 minutes. Add the kale and vegetable mixture and stir. Cook for 5-7 minutes, stirring occasionally. Add the spice blend and stir. Add the chickpeas and stir, cooking for 1 final minute.

TO ASSEMBLE: Spread the tzatziki sauce on the flatbread, layer the vegetable mix next, then top it off with the tahini sauce. Fold in half and enjoy right away or follow the trail instructions in the recipe introduction.

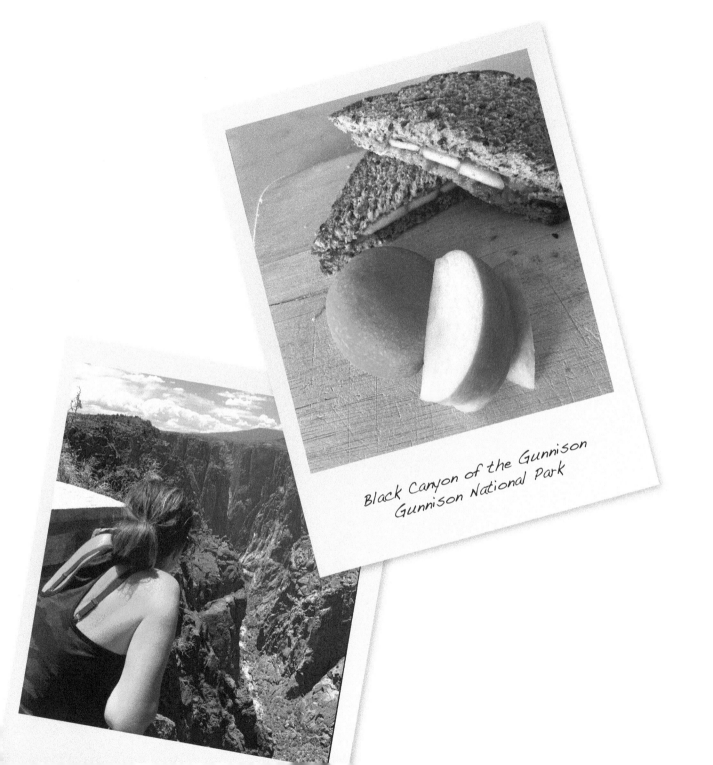

Black Canyon of the Gunnison
Gunnison National Park

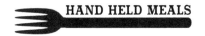

ELEVATED PB & J

I'm going back on my words about ditching the PB & J for a hike – all it needs is a little elevation to set it apart from the traditional standard. When we only have time for something very quick and easy, this is a great option. Choose a bread that is freshly made and really good quality, maybe from your local bakery or favorite market. The cinnamon and sliced apples make it special and a treat for your hike.

PREP TIME: 5 minutes
TOTAL TIME: 5 minutes
SERVES: 2

INGREDIENTS
4 slices of bread
2 TBS. peanut butter (or other nut, seed or nut-free butter)
2 TBS. strawberry jam (or other variety)
1 medium apple (any variety you like), thinly sliced
1 tsp. hemp hearts
Pinch cinnamon

DIRECTIONS
Spread one slice of bread with 1 TBS. nut butter and the other slice with 1 TBS. of the jam. Place a few of the apples on one slice, and sprinkle the pinch of cinnamon and half of the hemp hearts on the other. Assemble sandwich. Cut in half, if desired. Repeat with the other bread slices. Wrap in a sturdy container for toting to the trail so it keeps its shape and stays fresh.

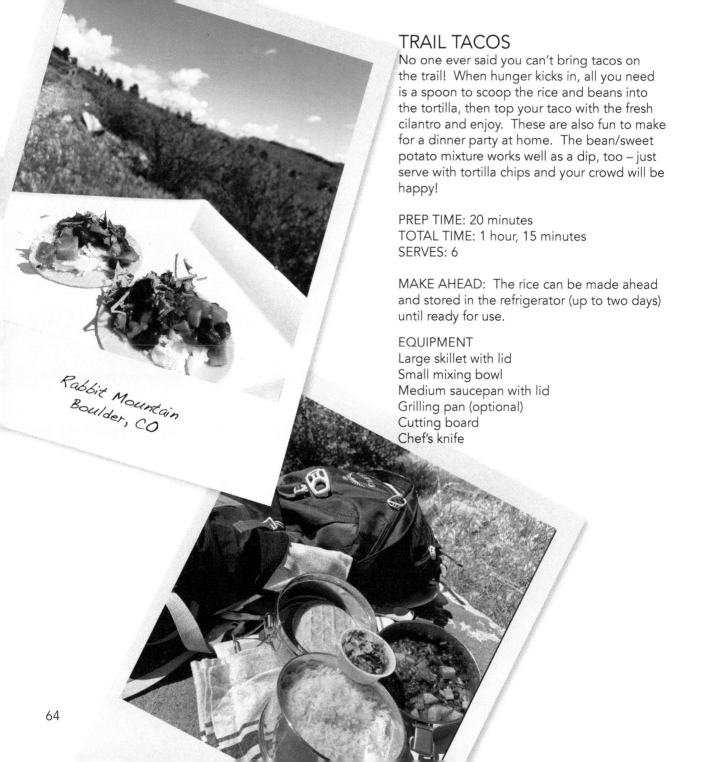

TRAIL TACOS

No one ever said you can't bring tacos on the trail! When hunger kicks in, all you need is a spoon to scoop the rice and beans into the tortilla, then top your taco with the fresh cilantro and enjoy. These are also fun to make for a dinner party at home. The bean/sweet potato mixture works well as a dip, too – just serve with tortilla chips and your crowd will be happy!

PREP TIME: 20 minutes
TOTAL TIME: 1 hour, 15 minutes
SERVES: 6

MAKE AHEAD: The rice can be made ahead and stored in the refrigerator (up to two days) until ready for use.

EQUIPMENT
Large skillet with lid
Small mixing bowl
Medium saucepan with lid
Grilling pan (optional)
Cutting board
Chef's knife

Rabbit Mountain
Boulder, CO

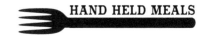

INGREDIENTS
¼ C. olive oil
1 medium onion, diced
5 garlic cloves, minced
1 shallot, diced
1 jalapeño pepper (optional), with or without seeds, diced
Spice blend (see recipe below)
1 medium sweet potato
(or other root vegetable variety), peeled and cubed

2 cans of black beans (NOT drained or rinsed)
½ C. water
1 bay leaf
1 TBS. apple cider vinegar
½ lime, squeezed
Fresh cilantro (about 1 tsp. to 1 TBS. per taco, chopped)
Long grain white rice (recipe below)
6 corn tortillas (or other tortilla variety)

SPICE BLEND
1 tsp. ground cumin
2 tsp. salt
1 tsp. oregano
½ tsp. ground black pepper
½ tsp. smoked paprika
Combine all spice blend ingredients in the small bowl, stir and set aside.

WHITE RICE
1 C. dry long grain white rice (such as basmati)
2 C. water
Pinch of salt
In the medium saucepan add the water and salt and bring to a rapid boil. Add the rice, stir and cover with the lid. Reduce heat to low and simmer for 15-20 minutes, until the water is absorbed. Try not to peek during the cooking time. Turn off the heat/remove from heat source and let sit, covered, for 5-10 minutes. Fluff the rice with a fork.

DIRECTIONS
Heat oil in skillet. Add onion and cook until soft, 2-3 minutes. Add garlic, shallot and jalapeños and stir, then cook for 2 minutes. Add the spice blend and stir, then cook for 1 minute. Add sweet potato, beans, water, bay leaf and vinegar and stir. Bring to a boil then turn the heat down to low. Cover and cook for 45-50 minutes. Remove the bay leaf. Add lime juice and adjust seasonings as needed. Scoop rice then beans into the tortilla. Top with chopped fresh cilantro.

TIP: If you like, grill the tortillas – it adds a yummy, smoky flavor. Lightly grease a grill pan or skillet and turn the heat on to medium. When heated, add as many tortillas as the skillet can hold without overlapping. When lightly golden brown grill marks appear, flip and grill the other side.

CALZONES WITH ROASTED VEGETABLES

Roasted vegetables in a pizza dough wrap is a simple dish to pack and eat with hand-held ease. These calzones can be customized individually – with picky eaters at my house, it's nice to have them made specially for each family member. And since the dough and sauce are ready made, that means less time in the kitchen! Before packing for your hike, heat the calzone then wrap in foil. Place in an insulated bag to help keep it warm for your trek out into nature.

PREP TIME: 45 minutes
TOTAL TIME: 1 hour, 15 minutes
MAKES: 4 calzones

EQUIPMENT
Baking sheet lined with parchment paper
Large mixing bowl
Cutting board
Chef's knife

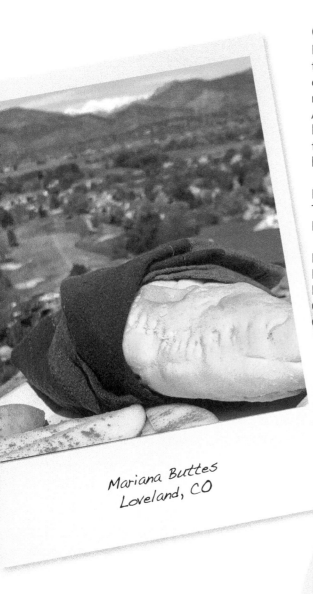

Mariana Buttes
Loveland, CO

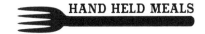

INGREDIENTS
1 pizza dough ball (ready made from the grocery store refrigerated section – take out of the fridge and thaw 30 minutes or until the dough comes to room temperature)
1-2 TBS. all-purpose flour (to prevent sticking)
1 can/jar of pizza sauce (look for organic or all-natural ingredients)
Spice blend (see recipe below)
Roasted vegetables (see recipe below)
1 C. nondairy mozzarella

SPICE BLEND
1 tsp. salt
½ tsp. pepper
1 tsp. oregano
Combine all spice blend ingredients in the small bowl, stir and set aside.

ROASTED VEGETABLES
2 TBS. olive oil
2 medium carrots, peeled and cut lengthwise
2 C. small broccoli florets
1 small red bell pepper, core removed and sliced lengthwise
1 jalapeño (optional) with or without seeds, trimmed and sliced lengthwise
Preheat the oven to 400°. In the large mixing bowl, add the olive oil and spice blend and stir until blended. Add the vegetables and mix until they're fully coated with the oil and spices. Spread them evenly on a baking sheet and place in the oven. Cook for 30 minutes, stirring halfway. Take out of the oven and set aside. Keep the oven temperature set at 400°.

DIRECTIONS
Divide the pizza dough into 4 equal sections. On a clean and floured surface, use your hands to work each section of dough, one at a time, to create a flattened circle (about 6" or so). On half the dough circle add the pizza sauce (start with a couple tablespoons and add more if desired), the roasted vegetables and 2 TBS. of the nondairy mozzarella cheese. Fold the dough in half and secure the edges by pressing down with your fingers or a fork to create a seal. Arrange the calzones on the baking sheet and bake (400°) for 30 minutes. Allow 5 minutes to cool, then enjoy. If eating later, cool completely then store covered or wrapped in foil in the refrigerator.

To reheat: Preheat oven to 350°. Place calzone wrapped in foil on a baking sheet in the oven for 20-25 minutes.

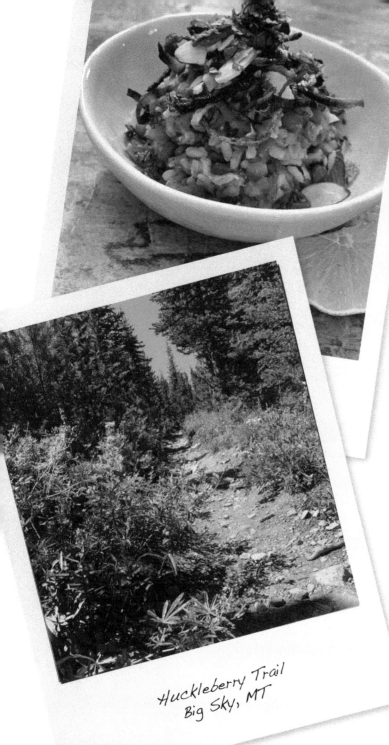

Huckleberry Trail
Big Sky, MT

MUJADARA WRAP

Here's a take on a traditional Middle Eastern concoction with za'atar seasoning and crispy onions on top – one of my very favorites! Stuff it all neatly into a tortilla and it can go anywhere with you.

PREP TIME: 1 hour
TOTAL TIME: 1 hour, 30 minutes
MAKES: 6 wraps

MAKE AHEAD: Toasted almonds and sliced onions can be prepared in advance. Store the toasted almonds in an airtight container in a cabinet or pantry, and the onions in an airtight container in the refrigerator – both for up to two days.

EQUIPMENT
Small mixing bowl
Baking sheet lined with parchment paper
2 medium saucepans with lids
Mandoline slicer (optional) or chef's knife
Cutting board
Large skillet or griddle

INGREDIENTS
1 C. brown basmati rice
2 bay leaves
2 C. water
½ C. green or brown lentils, rinsed
1 C. frozen riced cauliflower
1 ½ C. water
Spice blend (recipe, next page)
3 large yellow onions, thinly sliced
2 TBS. avocado oil
Toasted almonds (recipe, next page)
2 TBS. mint, chopped
Lettuce leaves, rinsed and patted dry
Squeeze of fresh lemon or lime juice
6 flour tortillas

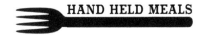

SPICE BLEND
4 tsp. za'atar seasoning – plus extra for finishing (OR 1 tsp. sesame seeds, 1 tsp. cumin,
1 tsp. chili powder, ½ tsp. salt, ½ tsp. garlic powder)
½ tsp. cayenne pepper (optional)
2 tsp. salt
Combine all spice blend ingredients in the small bowl, stir and set aside.

TOASTED ALMONDS
2 C. sliced almonds
Preheat oven to 350°. Place the almonds on a baking sheet. Bake for 4-5 minutes or until they are
golden brown and fragrant. Stay close by so they don't burn! Set aside to cool.

DIRECTIONS
In the medium saucepan, bring 2 C. water to a rapid boil then add the rice and bay leaves and give it
a quick stir. Cover, reduce heat to low and simmer for 40 minutes. Check to see if rice is fully cooked
and the water has been absorbed it may need a few additional minutes. Turn off the heat/remove
from heat source and set aside.

While the rice is cooking add the green lentils, water, riced cauliflower and spice blend in the other
saucepan. Bring to a boil then simmer, uncovered, for 20-25 minutes. Check lentils and cauliflower to
make sure they are soft (but not mushy), then drain and add to the saucepan with the rice. Stir, cover
and set aside.

While the rice and lentils/cauliflower are cooking, prep the onions by slicing them very thin manually
or use a mandoline to make the slicing go faster. Add the oil to the skillet on medium to medium
high heat. When heated add the sliced onions to the skillet (you may need to do 2 batches if you
don't have an extra-large pan). Allow the onions to get very crispy – that could take anywhere from
25-40 minutes, depending on how thinly they are sliced. Keep an eye on them and when crispy,
transfer to a plate lined with a paper towel. Put them aside until lentils and rice are cooked.

Transfer the rice/lentils/cauliflower mixture to the large mixing bowl. Add most of the crispy onions,
reserving some for the garnish. Stir gently.

PLATING
Heap a hearty scoop of the rice/lentil/cauliflower/onion mixture onto the tortilla. Top with the toasted
almonds, some remaining crispy onions, chopped herbs, lettuce, a small drizzle of olive oil, a sprinkle
of za'atar and/or cayenne and a squeeze of fresh lemon or lime juice.

TRAIL MIX SALAD

Kale is a cruciferous superhero packed with vitamins, minerals and antioxidants to help prevent and fight disease. Paired with the fresh punch of citrus from the lemon zest, sweetness of the blueberries and apple and crunch from the nuts and seeds is what gives this superfood so much personality. This trail mix inspired salad travels well in an airtight container and insulated bag ready to go with you on your journey.

PREP TIME: 15 minutes
TOTAL TIME: 2 hours 15 minutes
SERVES: 2

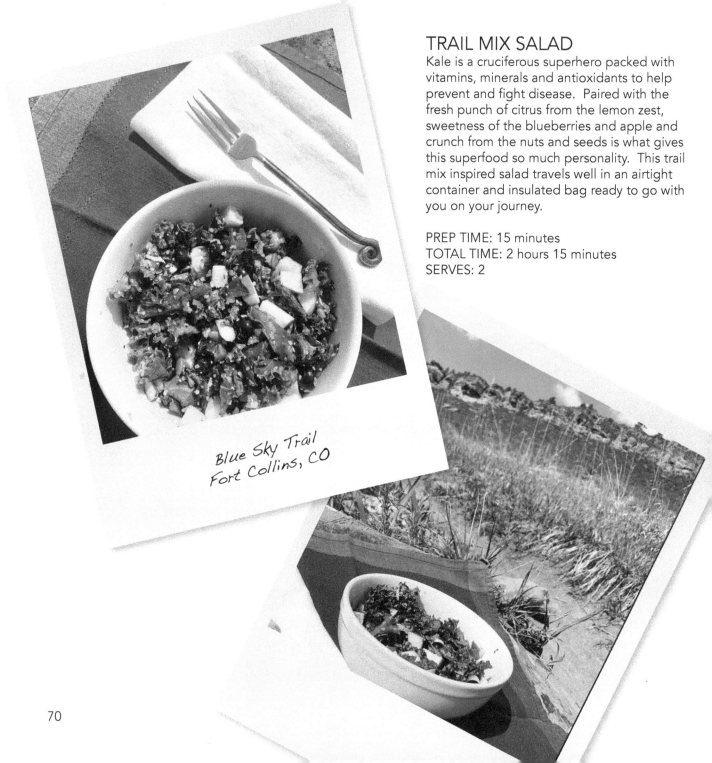

Blue Sky Trail
Fort Collins, CO

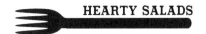

EQUIPMENT
Medium mixing bowl
Small mixing bowl
Whisk
Zester

INGREDIENTS
Trail Mix Salad Dressing (recipe below)
4 C. kale, rinsed, trimmed and cut into small bite-sized pieces
¼ C. hemp seeds
¼ C. pepitas (raw or roasted/salted)
¼ C. almonds (raw or roasted/salted)
¼ C. sunflower seeds (raw or roasted/salted)
1 medium crisp apple, cut into small cubes
1 C. fresh blueberries
Lemon zest

TRAIL MIX SALAD DRESSING
¼ C. olive oil
1 TBS. apple cider vinegar
1 tsp. dijon mustard
2 tsp. red onion, minced
1 TBS. pure maple syrup
1 pinch of salt
In the medium bowl, add the oil, vinegar, mustard, onion, maple syrup and salt and whisk until well blended. Add the kale and massage with hands for a minute or so until it's evenly distributed and the kale begins to break down. Cover and marinate in the fridge for at least 2 hours or overnight.

DIRECTIONS
In the small bowl, place the hemp seeds, pepitas, almonds, and sunflower seeds, stir and set aside. Remove the kale out from the fridge. Add the apples and blueberries. Add the seeds and nuts, and finish it off with the grated lemon zest, as much as you like. Mix the salad together gently until all the ingredients are evenly distributed. Enjoy right away or refrigerate for up to 2 days.

MUNG BEAN SALAD WITH SWISS CHARD

This simple salad is a refreshing change – especially if you've never tried healthy and delicious mung beans. Just one cup of these little green legumes has 14 grams of protein! I love the addition of the swiss chard, tomatoes and homemade red wine vinaigrette. This salad makes a wonderful side dish, or pair it with soup or a sandwich for a very comforting meal. Easy and portable in an airtight container – it can go right from the refrigerator to your backpack.

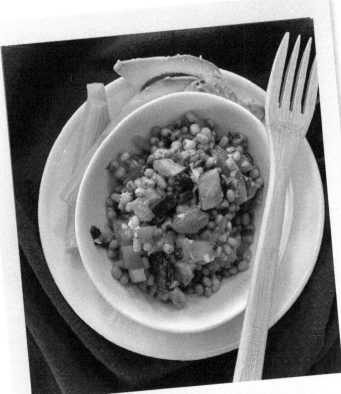

Fossil Creek Wetlands Natural Area
Fort Collins, CO

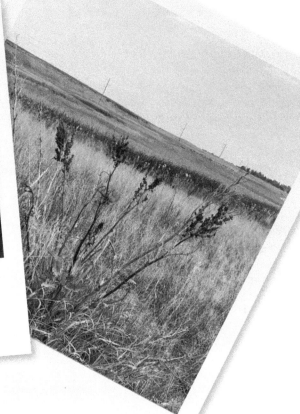

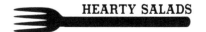

PREP TIME: 1 hour, 15 minutes
TOTAL TIME: 1 hour, 45 minutes
MAKES: 2 ½ cups

EQUIPMENT
Medium saucepan with lid
Large mixing bowl
Medium mixing bowl
Whisk
Colander
Cutting board
Chef's knife

INGREDIENTS
1 C. dry mung beans, soaked for at least an hour (or overnight) in water then drained
3 C. vegetable broth
2 C. tomatoes, diced
1 C. Swiss chard (or other power green such as kale or collards), roughly chopped
Red wine vinaigrette (recipe below)

RED WINE VINAIGRETTE
½ C. olive oil
3 TBS. red wine vinegar
1 tsp. Dijon mustard
1 clove fresh garlic, finely minced
1 tsp. dried oregano
Salt and pepper to taste
In a medium bowl, add all the ingredients and whisk until well blended.

DIRECTIONS
Place the soaked and drained mung beans in the saucepan with the vegetable broth. Bring to a boil then turn down the heat to low. Cover and cook for 30 minutes. Before removing from heat, check to see if the beans are fully cooked (but not mushy). They may need additional cooking time (this depends on how long they soak). Once cooked, drain in the colander and cool to room temperature. In the large bowl add the beans, tomatoes, chard and vinaigrette. Stir gently and serve right away or cover and refrigerate for up to 3 days.

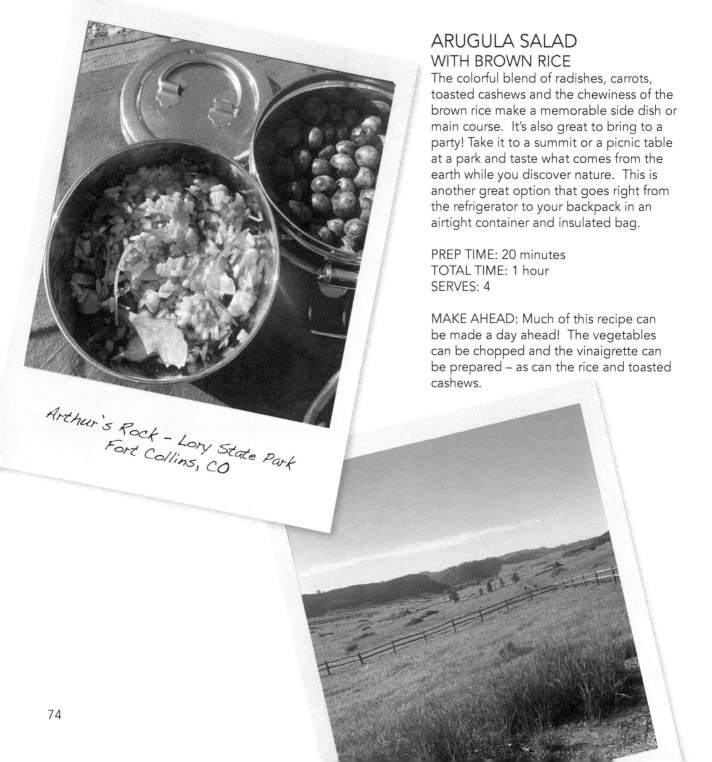

ARUGULA SALAD
WITH BROWN RICE

The colorful blend of radishes, carrots, toasted cashews and the chewiness of the brown rice make a memorable side dish or main course. It's also great to bring to a party! Take it to a summit or a picnic table at a park and taste what comes from the earth while you discover nature. This is another great option that goes right from the refrigerator to your backpack in an airtight container and insulated bag.

PREP TIME: 20 minutes
TOTAL TIME: 1 hour
SERVES: 4

MAKE AHEAD: Much of this recipe can be made a day ahead! The vegetables can be chopped and the vinaigrette can be prepared – as can the rice and toasted cashews.

Arthur's Rock - Lory State Park
Fort Collins, CO

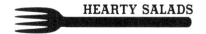

EQUIPMENT
Medium saucepan with lid
Large mixing bowl
Medium mixing bowl
Whisk
Cutting board
Chef's knife
Baking sheet lined with parchment paper

INGREDIENTS
1 C. dry brown rice
2 C. water
1/2 tsp. salt
6 C. arugula salad
1 C. carrots (orange or multi color), chopped
1 C. radishes, chopped
Toasted cashews (recipe below)
Red wine vinaigrette (recipe below)

RED WINE VINAIGRETTE
½ C. olive oil
3 TBS. red wine vinegar
1 tsp. Dijon mustard
1 clove fresh garlic, finely minced
1 tsp. dried oregano
Salt and pepper to taste
In the medium mixing bowl, add all the ingredients and whisk until well blended.

TOASTED CASHEWS
1 C. raw cashews
Preheat oven to 350°. Place nuts on the baking sheet and bake for 5 minutes or until golden brown and fragrant. They may need another minute or two of cooking time. Keep a close eye as they can burn easily. Allow to cool, then chop the cashews in large pieces and set aside.

DIRECTIONS
In the medium saucepan, add the rice, water and salt and bring to a boil. Cover and turn heat to low and simmer for 40-45 minutes. Turn off heat/remove from heat source, cover and let it sit for 5 minutes. Fluff with a fork and let it cool completely. In the large mixing bowl add the arugula, carrots, radishes and rice and stir. Add the dressing (start with half the dressing, then taste and add more if desired) and stir. Fold in the cashews. Enjoy right away or store in an airtight container for up to 2 days.

GREEK ORZO PASTA SALAD

This Mediterranean inspired salad is full of vegetables, hearty beans, orzo pasta and a vinaigrette with a touch of tahini (ground sesame seeds available at your local grocery store) added for creaminess. This is a favorite because it can go right from the refrigerator to a container and head straight for the trail. It's also an amazing main or side dish at home or to bring to a pot luck style gathering.

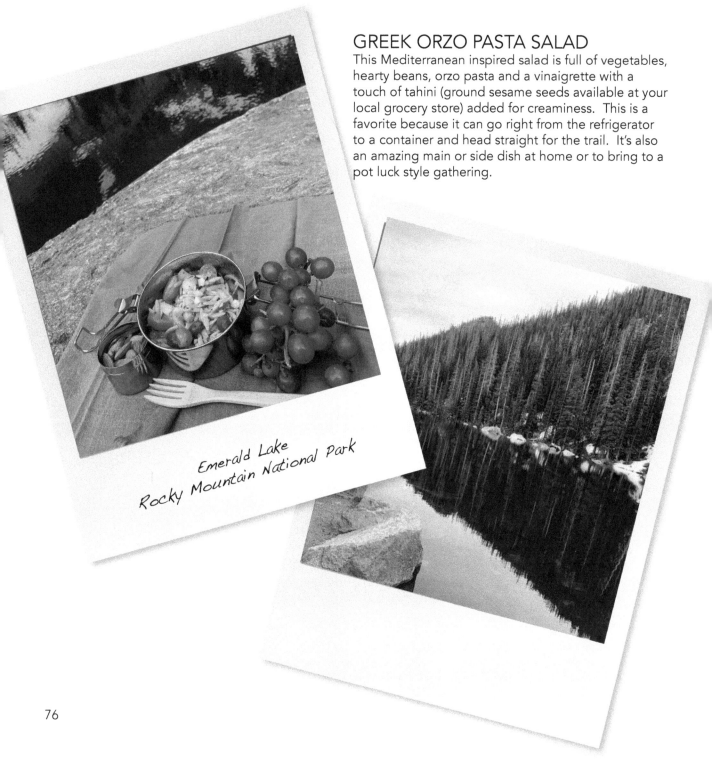

Emerald Lake
Rocky Mountain National Park

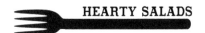
PREP TIME: 25 minutes
TOTAL TIME: 45 minutes
SERVES: 4-6

MAKE AHEAD: The vegetables can be prepared and stored in the refrigerator and the vinaigrette can be made the day before.

EQUIPMENT
Large saucepan with lid
Colander
Cutting board
Chef's knife
Large mixing bowl
Whisk

INGREDIENTS
2 C. water
¼ tsp. salt
1 C. dry orzo pasta
Red wine and tahini vinaigrette (recipe below)
1 can of chickpeas, drained and rinsed

1 C. kalamata olives
1 C. grape tomatoes, sliced in half
½ red onion, thinly sliced
1 C. cucumber, chopped
½ fresh lemon, squeezed
Salt to taste
2 C. fresh parsley, chopped

RED WINE AND TAHINI VINAIGRETTE
½ C. olive oil
1 TBS. tahini
3 TBS. red wine vinegar
1 tsp. Dijon mustard
1 clove fresh garlic, finely minced
1 tsp. dried oregano
Salt and pepper to taste
In the large mixing bowl, add all the ingredients and whisk until well blended.

DIRECTIONS
Add the water and salt to the saucepan on high and bring to a boil. Add the orzo, stir and cover. Reduce the heat and simmer for 8-10 minutes, until it is al dente. Drain and allow to cool down to room temperature. In the large mixing bowl (with the vinaigrette) add the cooked and cooled orzo pasta, chickpeas, olives, tomatoes, onion, and cucumber. Stir gently until all ingredients are coated with the dressing.   Top with the fresh lemon juice, salt and parsley. Enjoy right away or may be refrigerated for up to 3 days.

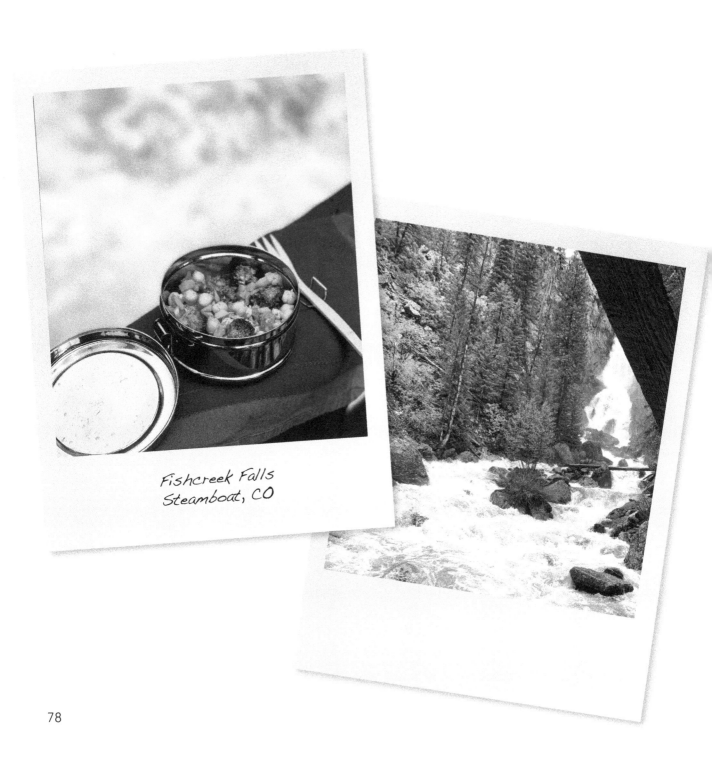

Fishcreek Falls
Steamboat, CO

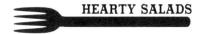

FARMERS MARKET SALAD

Thank you, Jody Jones, for passing along this recipe! Locally sourced ingredients from a farmers market or grocery store for this salad, combined with the tangy salad dressing (with smoked paprika!) is a wonderful way to enjoy a big serving vegetables. Loaded with nutrients that fuel and protect your body all in one bowl – plus it tastes amazing? Yes, please! So easy to pack up in an airtight container for the trail. Find a good spot and enjoy your veggies!

PREP TIME: 20 minutes
TOTAL TIME: 25 minutes
SERVES: 4-6

EQUIPMENT
Large mixing bowl
Cutting board
Sharp chef's knife
Medium mixing bowl
Whisk

INGREDIENTS
1 can of beans (any variety) drained and rinsed
½ C. red onion, diced
1 small red bell pepper, chopped
1 small yellow pepper, chopped

1 small head of broccoli, chopped
1 C. shredded carrots
Farmers Market Salad dressing
(see recipe below)

FARMERS MARKET SALAD DRESSING
½ C. olive oil
3 TBS. apple cider vinegar
½ tsp. smoked paprika (or regular paprika)
¼ tsp. garlic powder
1 tsp. oregano
1 tsp. maple syrup
Juice from ½ lemon
Salt and pepper to taste
In the medium bowl, add all ingredients and whisk until blended and set aside.

DIRECTIONS
Combine the beans and vegetables in the large mixing bowl and stir. Pour the dressing over the vegetable and bean mixture and stir until evenly coated. Cover and let marinate for an hour or overnight. Refrigerate for up to 3 days.

PEARLED BARLEY
WITH ORANGE VINAIGRETTE

The pearled barley combined with radishes and carrots is chewy, crisp and satisfying. This could be a wonderful side dish or a great main meal using a larger portion. The orange vinaigrette adds a citrus punch of flavor and the pearled barley has many nutritional benefits, including lots of dietary fiber. I imagine making a pit stop near a ponderosa pine grove to dig into this salad – the trees adding comforting shade on a sunny day.

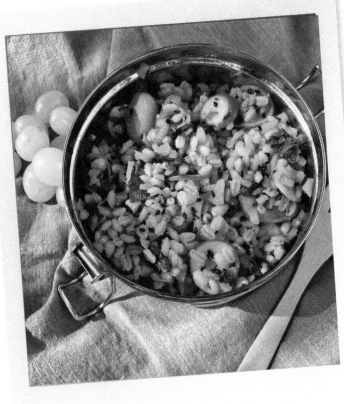

Flatirons Vista Trailhead
Boulder, CO

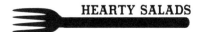

PREP TIME: 15 minutes
TOTAL TIME: 50 minutes
SERVES: 3

EQUIPMENT:
Large saucepan
Cutting board
Chef's knife
Colander
Large mixing bowl
Medium mixing bowl
Whisk

INGREDIENTS
8 C. water
1 C. uncooked pearled barley, rinsed
Pinch of salt
1 C. radishes, thinly sliced
1 C. carrots, chopped
1 C. cilantro, chopped (or other herb, or spinach)
2 TBS. black sesame seeds
Orange vinaigrette (recipe below)

ORANGE VINAIGRETTE
¼ C. orange juice
½ C. olive oil
¼ C. rice vinegar
Pinch of salt
Pinch of pepper
In the medium bowl, add all ingredients, whisk until well blended and set aside.

DIRECTIONS
Add the water and salt to the saucepan and set on high heat. When the water boils, add the barley and stir. Return to a boil and reduce the heat to medium. Cook for 25-30 minutes (uncovered). Test after 25 minutes of cooking to see if the barley is tender-chewy; cook for a few more minutes if not. Drain the excess water and run cold water over the barley until it's cooled. In the large mixing bowl, add the radishes, carrots, cilantro and sesame seeds. Add the orange vinaigrette (start with half the vinaigrette, then taste and add more if desired) and stir. Fold in the barley. Taste and add salt or pepper as needed. Serve right away, or cover and refrigerate up to 3 days.

COUSCOUS WITH TOASTED ALMONDS

This is one of those meals that takes very little time and provides so much in return. The couscous is fluffy and filling with the nutritional benefits and vibrant green color of kale. Top with a touch of olive oil and crunchy toasted almonds, and you'll complete a meal rich in flavor that's easy to pack up and take on the trail. The wildflowers, mountain view and fresh air are often my company for this meal and make it an even more memorable and tasty experience.

PREP TIME: 10 minutes
TOTAL TIME: 20 minutes
Serves: 2-3

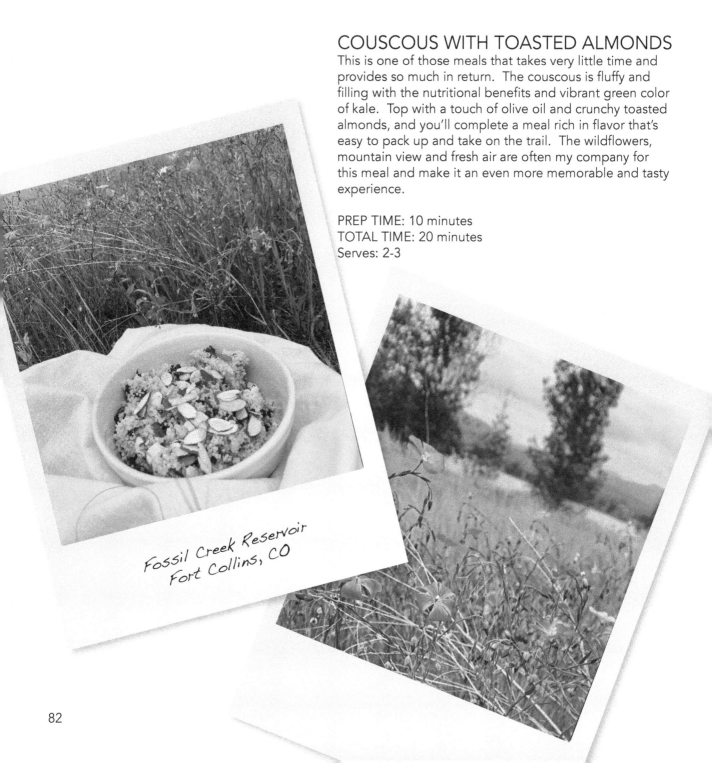

Fossil Creek Reservoir
Fort Collins, CO

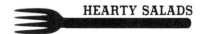

MAKE AHEAD: The toasted almonds can be made in advance – if you make extra, you'll have some on hand for salads, wraps, oatmeal and more.

EQUIPMENT
1 medium saucepan with lid
Baking sheet lined with parchment paper
Small mixing bowl
Cutting board
Chef's knife

INGREDIENTS
1 ½ C. water
2 tsp. olive oil (plus extra when finished)
½ C. chopped fresh kale
Spice blend (recipe below)
1 C. dry couscous, rinsed
Toasted almonds (recipe below)

SPICE BLEND
1 tsp. salt
1 tsp. oregano
1 tsp. garlic powder
½ tsp. red pepper flakes (optional)
Combine all spice blend ingredients in the small bowl, stir and set aside.

TOASTED ALMONDS
1 C. sliced almonds (plus more if you want leftovers)
Preheat oven to 350°. Place the almonds on a baking sheet and put in the oven for 5 minutes, or until they are just slightly golden. Keep a close eye since they can burn easily. Remove from the oven and set aside to cool completely. Leftover almonds can be stored in an airtight container in the pantry.

DIRECTIONS
In the medium saucepan, add water, oil, kale and spice blend. Stir, then bring to a boil. Add couscous, stir, cover, then turn off the heat/remove from heat source. Allow the couscous to sit for 10 minutes in the covered pot. When timer goes off, fluff with a fork. Allow to cool (or serve warm right away) and top with a drizzle of olive oil and toasted sliced almonds. If enjoying later, store in an airtight container and refrigerate up to 3 days.

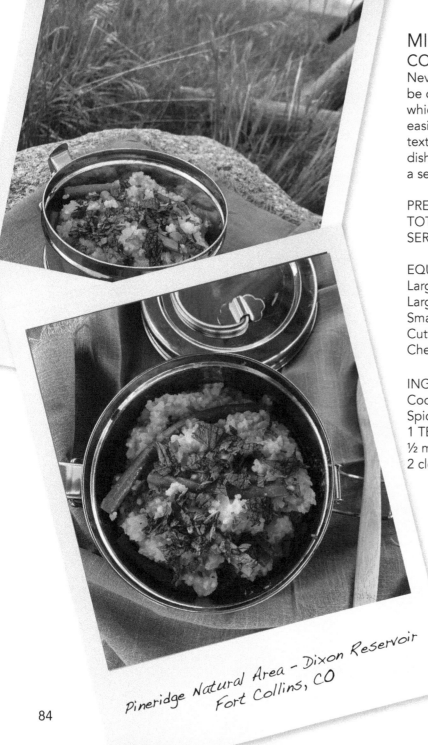

Pineridge Natural Area – Dixon Reservoir
Fort Collins, CO

MILLET WITH GREEN BEANS, COCONUT MILK AND TURMERIC

Never cooked with millet before? You won't be disappointed in this "ancient" grain – which means, among other things, it's more easily digestible – that has a soft and fluffy texture. To rev up the spice level of this dish, pick a pepper with more heat, such as a serrano or habañero.

PREP TIME: 30 minutes
TOTAL TIME: 1 hour
SERVES: 3

EQUIPMENT
Large saucepan with lid
Large deep skillet
Small mixing bowl
Cutting board
Chef's knife

INGREDIENTS
Cooked millet (recipe, next page)
Spice Blend (recipe, next page)
1 TBS. coconut oil
½ medium onion, diced
2 cloves garlic, minced

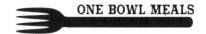

1 jalapeño pepper (optional), with or without seeds, diced
1 ½ C. fresh green beans, ends trimmed
1 medium red bell pepper, chopped
½ C. vegetable broth
1 C. coconut milk, full fat (freeze what is left)
One lime, cut in wedges
Salt and pepper to taste

COOKED MILLET
1 tsp. olive oil
1 C. dry millet
2 C. water
¼ tsp. salt
1 TBS. nondairy butter

Add olive oil to the large saucepan and bring to medium heat. Add the millet and toast for 4-5 minutes, stirring occasionally, until you can smell a nutty aroma. Add the water and salt; stir. Bring to a boil, then reduce the heat to low and add the butter and stir. Cover and simmer for 15 minutes, then turn the heat off/remove from heat source. Let stand covered for 10 minutes then fluff with a fork. Try to resist the temptation to lift the lid and peek during the cooking and standing process. While the millet is cooking, start the rest of the recipe.

SPICE BLEND
1 tsp. turmeric
1 tsp. ginger powder
1 tsp. salt
1 tsp. cumin
Combine all spice blend ingredients in the small bowl, stir and set aside.

DIRECTIONS
Add coconut oil to a large skillet and bring to medium heat. Add the onion and cook for 2-3 minutes, until soft. Add the garlic, jalapeño and spice blend. Stir and cook for 1 minute. Mix in the green beans, red pepper and vegetable broth. Cook for 3-4 minutes, or until the green beans are fork tender. Add the coconut milk and stir. Cook for 1-2 more minutes until the coconut milk is fully heated, just shy of a boil. Turn off the heat/remove from heat source. Add the cooked millet to the skillet and stir. Add the squeeze of lime juice – taste and add salt/pepper as needed. If making ahead for the trail, cool completely then store in the refrigerator for up to 3 days.

LEMONY PASTA AND PEAS

Peas and fresh lemon juice come together to add brightness and depth of flavor to this hike-friendly, whole-wheat pasta meal, which is made creamy with the healthy addition of nutty tahini. This dish is a bit heavier on oil, butter and salt so adjust as needed if you have dietary restrictions. Try this meal for dinner, then warm it up the next day and put into an airtight, insulated container (to keep it warm or room temp) for an enjoyable lunch on the trail.

PREP TIME: 25 minutes
TOTAL TIME: 45 minutes
SERVES: 6

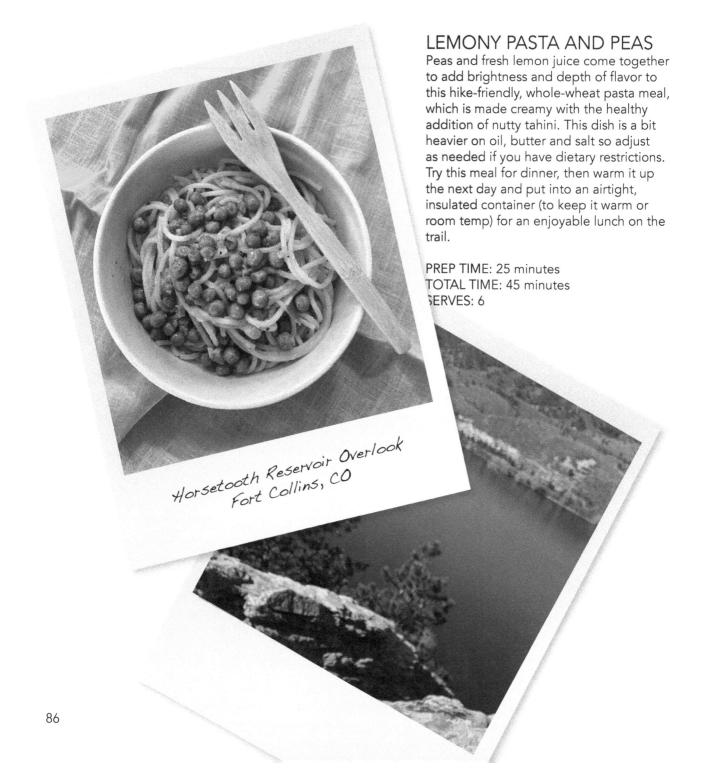

Horsetooth Reservoir Overlook
Fort Collins, CO

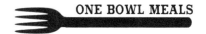

EQUIPMENT
Large saucepan with lid
Large skillet
Colander
Tongs
Cutting board
Chef's knife
Zester

INGREDIENTS
16 oz. whole wheat spaghetti (or other pasta of your liking)
5-6 quarts of water
1 tsp. salt
½ C. olive oil plus 1 TBS.
8 TBS. nondairy butter
2 shallots, minced
2 TBS. tahini
2 tsp. salt
½ tsp. red pepper flakes, optional
1 16 oz. bag of frozen or fresh peas
1 C. reserved pasta water
Handful of basil, cut into thin strips (julienned) or 1 tsp. dried basil
1 lemon, juiced
1 TBS. lemon zest
Nondairy parmesan cheese, grated (optional)
Nutritional yeast (optional)

DIRECTIONS
In the large saucepan bring the water and salt to a rolling boil. Add the spaghetti. Return to a boil, then reduce heat to low and simmer for 9-11 minutes, or until al dente, stirring occasionally. Drain in the colander and return to saucepan. Add 1 TBS. of olive oil to the spaghetti and stir. Cover and set aside while you are making the rest of the recipe. In the large skillet over medium heat, add the butter and ½ C. olive oil. Once heated, add the shallot and cook for 2-3 minutes, until soft. Add the tahini, salt and red pepper flakes and stir. Add the peas and reserved pasta water and cook 3-4 minutes (check the peas to make sure they are cooked thoroughly). Turn off the heat/remove from heat source. Add the spaghetti and combine it with the sauce. Fold in the basil and lemon juice with the tongs. Top with lemon zest and nondairy parmesan or a sprinkle of nutritional yeast.

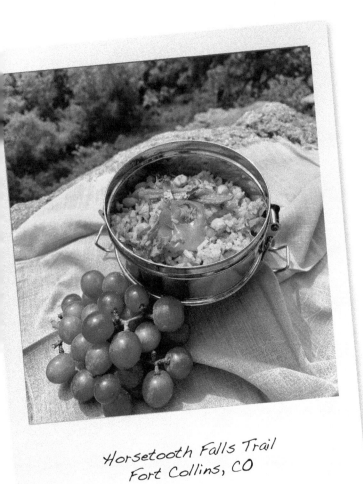

Horsetooth Falls Trail
Fort Collins, CO

AROUND THE WORLD FRIED RICE

Pick the world region's flavors you are craving and get cooking! The herb and nut garnishes can be swapped out for anything that sounds good to you – suggestions are included in the recipe, but don't let that stop your creativity. This dish might seem a bit heavier on the oil and salt, so if you are watching either or both of those, decide for yourself if you need to cut back. Your meal will still be delicious with less! For the trail, place in an airtight container and start your trek. Bring some fruit along to finish your meal with a little sweetness.

PREP TIME: 45
TOTAL TIME: 1 hour 15 minutes
SERVES: 4-6

EQUIPMENT
Baking sheet lined with parchment paper
Large saucepan with lid
Large skillet
Chef's knife
Cutting board

INGREDIENTS
1 C. toasted nuts (see spice blend recipes for suggestions, next page)
1 ½ C. dry basmati rice, rinsed (see recipe, next page)
3 TBS. coconut oil
2 hot peppers (jalapeño, serrano, habañero, etc.), seeds removed (or keep the seeds to increase the heat), sliced into thick strips
2-3 cloves of garlic, minced
3 C. mixed vegetables, chopped (red pepper, carrots and zucchini – or choose your own favorites)
Spice blend (see recipe on next page for variations)
Fresh herbs, chopped (see garnish tips, next page)
Squeeze of fresh lime juice

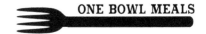

INDIAN SPICE BLEND
1 tsp. turmeric, 2 tsp. chili powder, 2 tsp. cumin seeds, ½ tsp. garam masala, ½ tsp. ground ginger, 1 ½ tsp. salt
Combine all spice blend ingredients in the small bowl, stir and set aside.
GARNISH TIP: chopped fresh mint and toasted raw cashews, toasted (toasted nut directions below)

MEXICAN SPICE BLEND
2 tsp. chili powder, 2 tsp. cumin, ½ tsp. dried oregano, ½ tsp. paprika, ½ tsp. garlic powder, ½ tsp. onion powder, 1 ½ tsp. salt
Combine all spice blend ingredients in the small bowl, stir and set aside.
GARNISH TIP: chopped fresh cilantro and roasted and salted pepitas

ASIAN SPICE BLEND
2 tsp. onion powder, 2 tsp. garlic powder, 1 tsp. ground ginger, 1 tsp. black pepper, ½ tsp. red pepper flakes, 4 tsp. sesame seeds, 1 ½ tsp. salt
Combine all spice blend ingredients in the small bowl, stir and set aside.
GARNISH TIP: chopped fresh cilantro and toasted raw peanuts (toasted nut directions below)

TOASTED NUTS
Preheat oven to 350. Place nuts on a baking sheet and put in the oven for about 5 minutes, or until they become fragrant and turn golden brown (they burn easily, keep an eye out towards the end of the cooking process). Set aside to cool.

BASMATI RICE
3 TBS. nondairy butter
1 ½ C. dry basmati rice
2 ¾ C. vegetable broth
Melt nondairy butter in the large saucepan over medium heat. Add the rice and stir occasionally, allowing the rice to toast for 5 minutes (this brings out the nutty, delicious flavor of the rice).
Add broth and stir. Bring to a boil then reduce heat and cover. Simmer for 15 minutes. Turn off heat/ remove from heat source and let sit, covered, for an additional 5 minutes. Fluff with fork, recover and set aside.

DIRECTIONS
Melt the coconut oil in the skillet over medium heat. When the oil has melted, add the pepper strips to the skillet and cook for 2-3 minutes, or until the skin on the pepper starts to blister. Add the garlic, stir and cook for 1 minute. Add the mixed vegetables and cook for 3-5 minutes or until fork tender (stirring occasionally). Turn off the heat/remove from heat source. Add the spice blend and stir, then fold in the cooked basmati rice. Ladle the fried rice onto a plate or into a bowl. Top with herbs and toasted nuts of choice, and a squeeze of fresh lime juice.

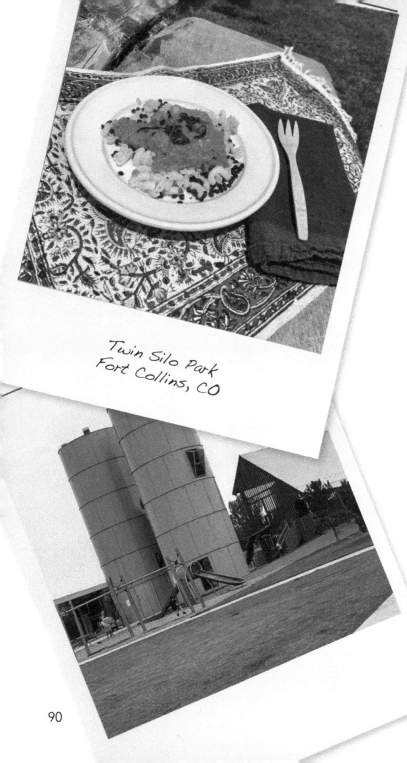

Twin Silo Park
Fort Collins, CO

KOSHARI

This national dish of Egypt recipe calls for some extra steps (the brown rice, lentils and macaroni are all cooked separately) but it's totally worth the effort. During this time in the kitchen I like to have other things to do like stretch, pay bills or catch up on reading. You can also make the pasta, rice and/or lentils the day before. The aroma of the onions frying in your kitchen is heaven! This meal sustains and is perfect for when your belly starts to rumble on the trail. Take this one on, I promise you'll love it.

PREP TIME: 2 hours
TOTAL TIME: 3 hours
SERVES: 6

EQUIPMENT
Small mixing bowl
3 medium saucepans (for the lentils, macaroni and rice – or cook individually, one at a time, with one saucepan)
Colander
Large skillet
Blender
Large bowl
Chef's knife
Cutting board

INGREDIENTS
1 C. brown rice (recipe, next page)
2 C. water
½ tsp. salt
½ C. beluga lentils, or green or brown lentils (rinse then pick over to remove agricultural debris. Recipe, next page)
1 ½ C. water
1 C. elbow macaroni (recipe, next page)
8 C. water
1 tsp. salt
3 TBS. avocado oil
2 large yellow onions, thinly sliced
2 large ripe tomatoes, diced

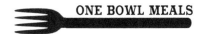

SPICE BLEND
2 tsp. cumin
2 tsp. garlic powder
1 tsp. chili powder
¼ - ½ tsp. red pepper flakes (to taste)
1 tsp. salt
Combine all ingredients in the small bowl and set aside.

BROWN RICE
In the medium saucepan, add the rice, water and salt and bring to a boil. Cover and turn heat to low, then simmer for 40-45 minutes. Turn off the heat, and set the rice aside.

LENTILS
In the medium saucepan, add the water and lentils. Bring to a boil, then cover and reduce heat to low for 20 minutes. Check to see if the lentils are cooked thoroughly (but not mushy). Turn off the heat. Drain excess water, if there is any, and put aside.

ELBOW MACARONI
In the medium saucepan, add the water and salt and bring to a boil. Add the macaroni, cover, and reduce heat to low for 7-9 minutes, or until pasta is al dente. Drain in a colander and put aside.

DIRECTIONS
In a large skillet, heat the oil to medium-high. Add the onions and cook until they are brown and crispy on the edges (you may need to do 2 batches if you don't have an extra-large pan). When they're done, take ¼ C. of the crispiest onions out of the pan and set aside – these will be used for a garnish on top of your koshari. Turn the heat down to medium, add the tomatoes and spices and stir. Cook for 20 minutes – you'll see the skin on the tomatoes start to curl (an additional few minutes may be needed). Once they are cooked down completely, turn off the heat and allow the mixture to cool. Once cooled, place the onion/tomato mixture into a blender and pulse until you have the consistency you desire (it can be smooth or chunky, it's up to you). Return the mixture to the skillet and turn the heat on to medium so the sauce can reheat. See the options below on how to plate this meal.

PLATING
Option 1: In the large bowl add the rice, lentils and macaroni (all heated/reheated) and stir, then top it off with the onion/tomato sauce.
Option 2: Heat/reheat the ingredients individually then layer the macaroni, lentils, brown rice and sauce like you would a lasagna. Either top with the reserved crispy onions and serve, or let your Koshari cool completely, then place in an airtight container and store in the refrigerator for up to 3 days.

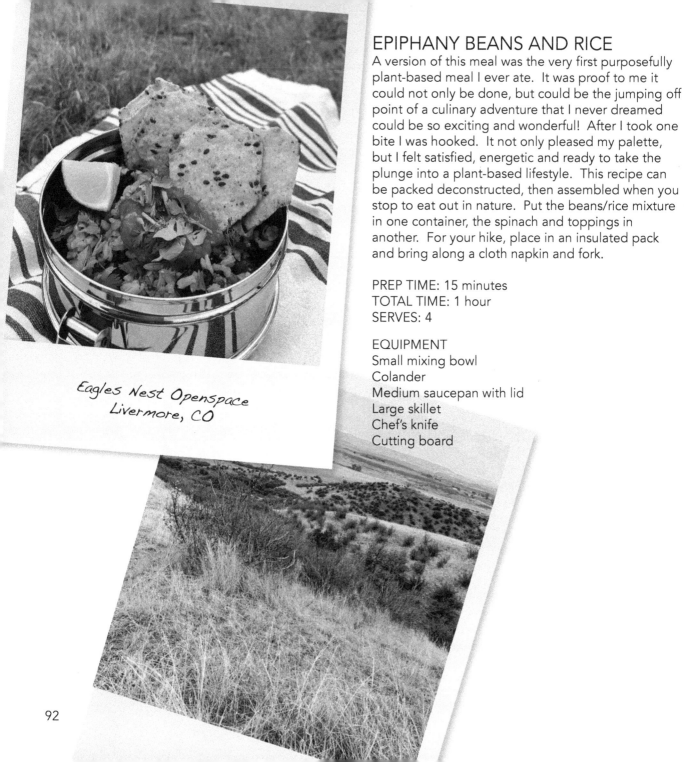

EPIPHANY BEANS AND RICE

A version of this meal was the very first purposefully plant-based meal I ever ate. It was proof to me it could not only be done, but could be the jumping off point of a culinary adventure that I never dreamed could be so exciting and wonderful! After I took one bite I was hooked. It not only pleased my palette, but I felt satisfied, energetic and ready to take the plunge into a plant-based lifestyle. This recipe can be packed deconstructed, then assembled when you stop to eat out in nature. Put the beans/rice mixture in one container, the spinach and toppings in another. For your hike, place in an insulated pack and bring along a cloth napkin and fork.

PREP TIME: 15 minutes
TOTAL TIME: 1 hour
SERVES: 4

EQUIPMENT
Small mixing bowl
Colander
Medium saucepan with lid
Large skillet
Chef's knife
Cutting board

Eagles Nest Openspace
Livermore, CO

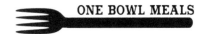

INGREDIENTS
1 C. brown rice, rinsed
2 C. water
½ tsp. salt
1 TBS. olive oil
½ C. onion, diced
2-3 cloves of garlic
1 jalapeño pepper (optional), with or without seeds, diced
Spice blend (see recipe below)
1 15 oz. can of black beans, drained and rinsed
Salt to taste
1 C. fresh spinach
Fresh cilantro, chopped
1 avocado, sliced
Salsa or hot sauce (optional)
Tortilla chips (optional)

SPICE BLEND
½ tsp. cumin
½ tsp oregano
½ tsp. salt
Combine all spice blend ingredients in the small bowl, stir and set aside.

BROWN RICE
In the medium saucepan, add the rice, water and salt and stir. Bring to a boil, then turn heat to low.
Cover and simmer for 40-45 minutes, until the rice is tender. Remove from heat source and set aside.

DIRECTIONS
Heat 1 TBS. olive oil in the skillet over medium heat. Add the onion, stir, and cook for 2-3 minutes
or until soft. Add the garlic and jalapeño, stir, then cook for 1 minute. Add the spice blend and stir.
Add the cooked rice and drained beans and mix together. When the mixture is thoroughly heated,
turn the heat off/remove from heat source. Taste to see if additional salt is needed. If serving right
away, scoop a generous portion of the bean/rice mixture onto a plate. Add ¼ cup spinach per
portion, then top with the sliced avocado, salsa (if using), cilantro and a handful of tortilla chips.

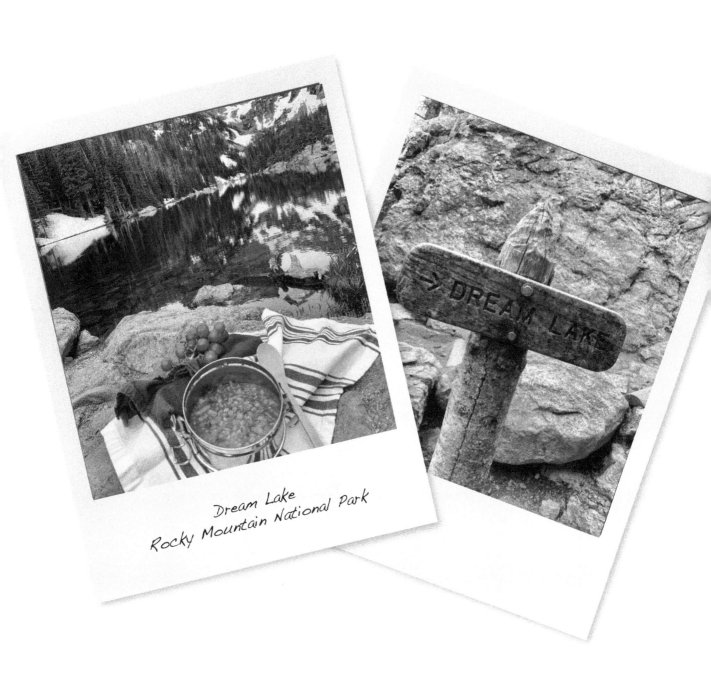

Dream Lake
Rocky Mountain National Park

DREAM LAKE

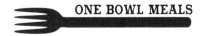

VEGETABLE SOUP WITH SMOKED PAPRIKA

Does preparing a favorite dish ever make you think of a loved one? When I make soup I am reminded of my dear friend Mimi Desta, one of the best cooks I've ever known. She owns a café in Fulton, Maryland called Sidamo Coffee and Tea. If you are ever lucky enough to be in the DC/Baltimore area – especially in the winter when she has soup on the menu – a visit to Sidamo will be worth the trip, I promise. This recipe calls for smoked paprika, a great replacement for standard paprika when you want to add a smoky and more intense attitude to your meal. It's widely available at many grocery stores and it adds so much extra flavor and depth! This soup should be packed up in an insulated container and an insulated bag to help retain the warm temperature of the stew for your day hike meal.

PREP TIME: 25 minutes
TOTAL TIME: 1 hour, 20 minutes
SERVES: 5

EQUIPMENT
Large saucepan
Chef's knife
Cutting board

INGREDIENTS
¼ C. olive oil
1 C. onion, chopped
1" fresh ginger, peeled and minced
1 jalapeño (optional), seeds or no seeds, diced
2-3 cloves of garlic, minced
½ of a 6 oz. can of tomato paste (save the other half and freeze it for future use)
½ tsp. smoked paprika
2 tsp. salt
2 C. carrots, sliced
1 C. red bell pepper, seeded and chopped
8 C. water
1 C. red lentils, rinsed
1 C. green lentils, rinsed
Fresh lemon juice from half a lemon
1 C. fresh herbs or greens (such as cilantro, kale or spinach), chopped

DIRECTIONS
Add olive oil to the saucepan on medium heat. Once heated, add the onion and cook until soft, about 2-3 minutes. Add ginger, jalapeño and garlic. Stir and cook 1 minute. Add the tomato paste, smoked paprika and salt and stir until fragrant, about 1 minute. Add the carrots and red bell pepper, stir and cook for 1 minute. Add the water and green and red lentils and stir. Bring to a strong boil then reduce heat to low and cover. Simmer for 45 minutes, then turn off the burner/remove from heat source. Add lemon juice and herbs/greens, then put the cover back on for 5 minutes (keep the heat off). Stir, taste and add salt if needed.

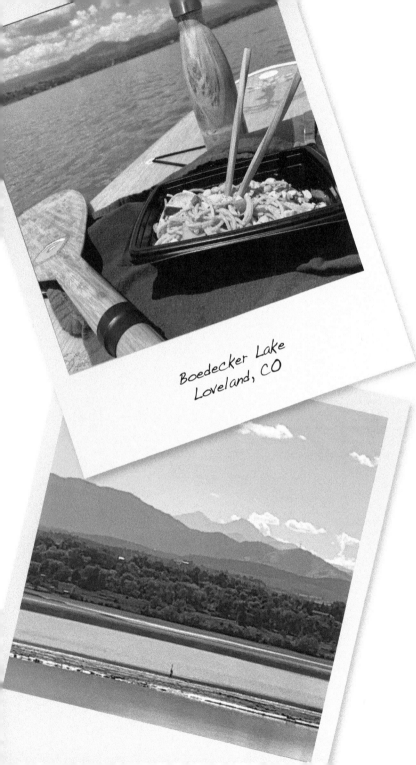

Boedecker Lake
Loveland, CO

PEANUT NOODLES
WITH VEGETABLES

I've been making this recipe – with so many variations – for many, many years. Swapping out vegetables and pastas is fun, and the dish is always good because the peanut sauce has so much flavor. For this pictured meal break, I found a quiet spot on the lake to enjoy the noodles. The slight rhythmic movement on the water, the rustling of the breeze in the trees on the shore and the sunshine made it taste extra special.

PREP TIME: 45 minutes
TOTAL TIME: 1 hour, 15 minutes
SERVES: 4

MAKE AHEAD: The peanut sauce can be made up to 3 days ahead. When ready to use, take out of the refrigerator and let it sit on the counter until it reaches room temperature.

EQUIPMENT
Cutting board
Chef's knife Blender
Baking sheet lined with parchment paper
Large saucepan
Colander
Large skillet
Tongs

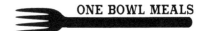

INGREDIENTS
1 16 oz. box of brown rice noodles
1 tsp. salt
5 quarts water
Peanut sauce (recipe below)
¼ C. toasted sesame oil
2 medium carrots, julienned
1 C. snow peas
1 red bell pepper, thinly sliced
2 green onions, thinly sliced (reserve green parts for garnish, save the rest for another recipe)
½ C. toasted peanuts, chopped (recipe below)
Lime wedges

PEANUT SAUCE
½ C. peanut butter
2 TBS. liquid aminos (or soy sauce, or soy sauce alternative)
1 TBS. rice vinegar
1 TBS. maple syrup
½ tsp. ginger powder
½ tsp. garlic powder
½ tsp. cayenne pepper
½ tsp. salt
½ C. water
¼ C. toasted sesame oil
In a blender, add the peanut butter, aminos, vinegar, maple syrup, ginger powder, garlic powder, cayenne pepper, salt, water and toasted sesame oil and blend until emulsified. Set aside.

TOASTED PEANUTS
Set oven to 350°. Place peanuts on a baking sheet and bake for 5 minutes or until lightly golden brown and fragrant. Cool, then chop into small crumbles.

DIRECTIONS
In the large saucepan, add the water and salt on high heat and bring to a boil. Add the noodles, stir, and return to a boil. Reduce the heat and simmer for 9-10 minutes, or until tender. Drain in a colander, rinse with cool water and set aside. Heat the toasted sesame oil in the skillet over medium heat. Add the carrots, snow peas and red bell pepper. Stir occasionally until tender-crisp, about 3-5 minutes. Turn off the heat. Add the noodles and peanut sauce to the skillet and mix together with tongs. Serve right away, or store in an airtight container and refrigerate up to 3 days. The noodles are delicious at room temperature or warmed up. Garnish with the green onions, peanuts and a fresh lime wedge.

TACO QUINOA
WITH PEANUTS AND KALE

Peanuts are a nice surprise in this taco-inspired recipe! Serve this dish in a soft tortilla wrap, or on a bed of lettuce (or spinach) with some chopped up vegetables and tortilla chips – there are many portable possibilities for consuming this on the trail.

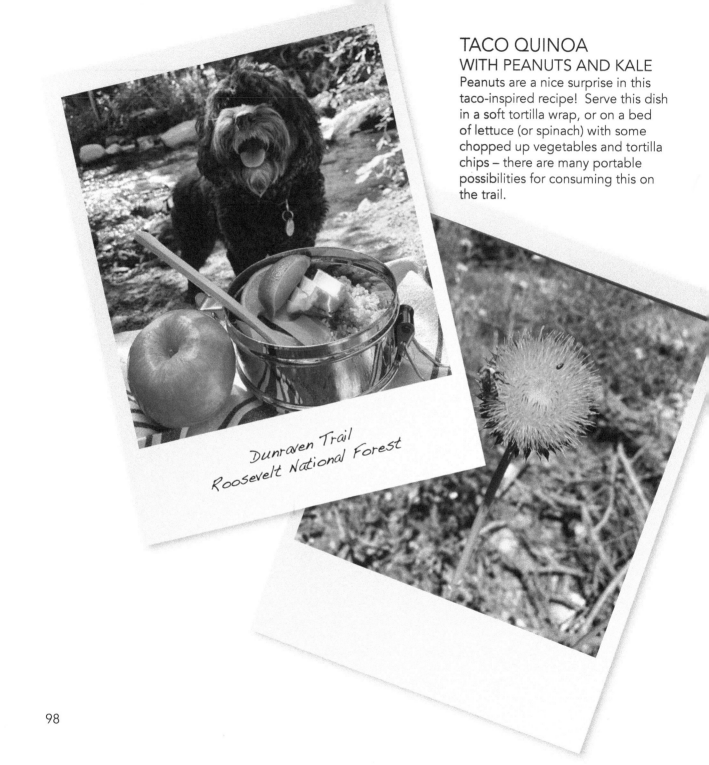

Dunraven Trail
Roosevelt National Forest

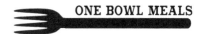

PREP TIME: 10 minutes
TOTAL TIME: 30 minutes
MAKES: 3 ½ - 4 cups

EQUIPMENT
Medium saucepan with lid
Cutting board
Chef's knife
Small mixing bowl

INGREDIENTS
1 C. dry quinoa (rinsed)
2 ¼ C. water
1 ½ C. kale, chopped
¾ C. peanuts (any variety - dry roasted, raw, blanched, etc.)
Spice blend (recipe below)
Avocado slices
Lime wedges

SPICE BLEND
1 tsp. oregano
1 tsp. garlic powder
1 tsp. onion powder
½ tsp. cumin
½ tsp. chili powder
½ tsp. salt
Pinch red pepper flakes (optional)
Combine all spice blend ingredients in the small bowl, stir and set aside.

DIRECTIONS
Place the quinoa, water, kale, peanuts and spice blend in the saucepan and stir. Turn the heat on high and bring to a boil. Then turn the heat down to low, cover and simmer for 15 minutes. Turn off the heat/remove from heat source, and let sit, covered, for 5 minutes. Fluff with a fork, then serve with the avocado slices and a squeeze of fresh lime juice. If preparing for a hike, allow to cool and place in an airtight container. Store in the fridge for up to 3 days.

TIP: When I bring a dish on a hike that features avocado, I bring a whole avocado and a small knife to cut it (don't forget a napkin to wrap the knife in after use). This way, you avoid browning and the avocado is fresh for your meal.

LEMON-BASIL PESTO PASTA

There will be plenty of extra pesto when you prepare this recipe – that's on purpose. Freeze what you don't use, and you will have pesto readily available for another time (and another trail!). Fresh tomatoes on the side compliment this dish wonderfully. The pasta and tomatoes can be packed together in one airtight container for the trail to save on space.

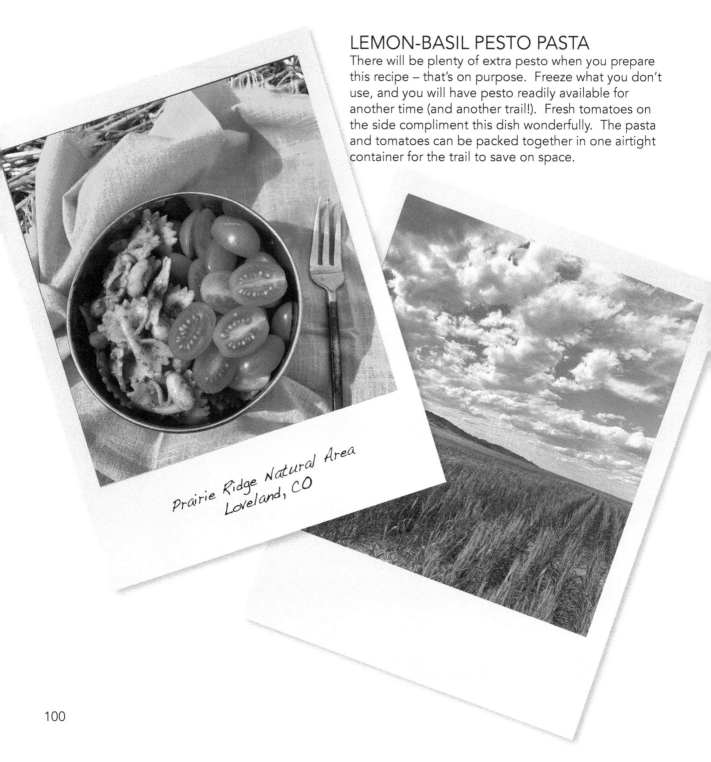

Prairie Ridge Natural Area
Loveland, CO

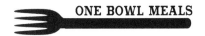

PREP TIME: 40 minutes
TOTAL TIME: 1 hour
SERVES: 3-4
MAKES: 1 ½ C. pesto (Save half and freeze for later. Leftovers can be packed into an ice cube tray or muffin tin to create individual servings!)

EQUIPMENT
Large saucepan
Colander
Large bowl
Blender
Cutting board
Chef's knife

INGREDIENTS
6 quarts water
½ tsp. salt
2 C. dry farfalle pasta
¾ C. Lemon-Basil Pesto (recipe below)
1 can of northern beans, drained and rinsed
2 C. grape or cherry tomatoes, sliced in half

LEMON-BASIL PESTO
4 C. loosely packed fresh basil
2 TBS. fresh oregano, chopped (or 1 tsp. dried)
¾ C. olive oil
½ C. roasted and salted pistachios
¼ C. pine nuts
1 TBS. hemp hearts
¼ tsp. red pepper flakes (optional)
½ tsp. salt
Juice of one lemon
Add all the ingredients to a blender and blend until smooth.

DIRECTIONS
In the large saucepan, bring 4 quarts of water and ½ tsp. salt to a boil. Add the farfalle, stir and return to a boil. Turn heat to low and simmer, uncovered, for 9-11 minutes, stirring occasionally. Drain in a colander. In the large bowl, add the pasta and half the pesto and stir. Add the beans and gently fold into the pasta/pesto mix. Allow time to cool to room temperature. Serve right away or place in the refrigerator for up to 3 days. When plating, add the tomatoes on the side.

ETHIOPIAN STYLE LENTILS

I enjoy these spicy and comforting lentils especially with fresh homemade flatbread (recipe P. 53) – it's perfect for dipping the delicious lentils and broth. No time? Not a problem! You can absolutely buy the flatbread ready made at the store – if you do, toast it and add a drizzle of olive oil and a sprinkle of salt just before eating. Crackers or tortilla chips are also a great option. This one-pot meal is simple to make and easy to pack and go – just put the lentils in an insulated container, wrap up the flatbread or chips and get out there!

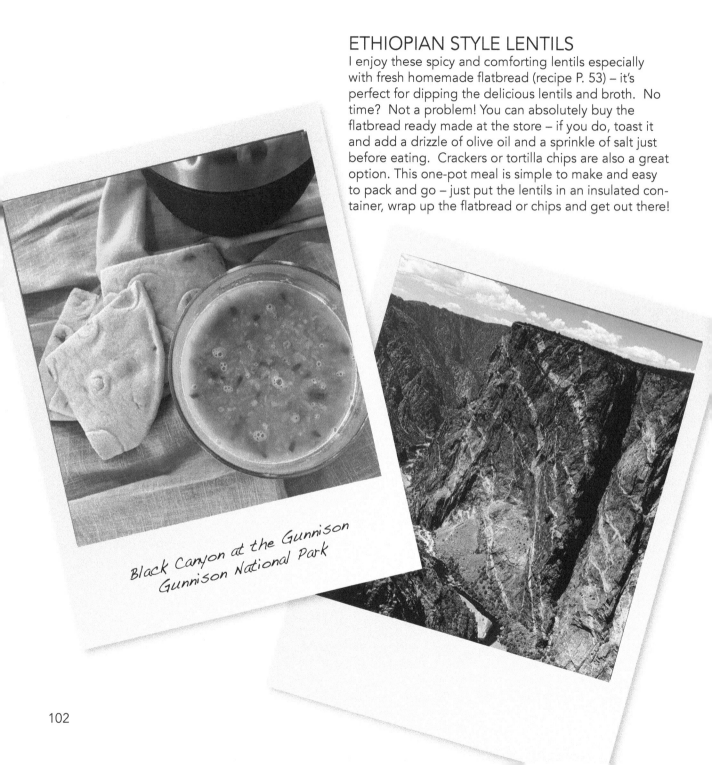

Black Canyon at the Gunnison
Gunnison National Park

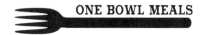

PREP TIME: 15 minutes
TOTAL TIME: 45 minutes
SERVES: 3

EQUIPMENT
Cutting board
Chef's knife
Medium saucepan with lid
Small mixing bowl (if using berbere seasoning substitute)

INGREDIENTS
½ C. olive oil
1 onion, chopped
2 cloves garlic, chopped
1 TBS. fresh ginger, chopped
1 large tomato, chopped
1 tsp. berbere seasoning or substitute (recipe below)
½ tsp. salt
2 ½ C. water
1 C. red lentils, rinsed
Salt, to taste
Fresh cilantro, chopped (optional)

BERBERE SEASONING SUBSTITUTE
¼ tsp. cayenne pepper
¼ tsp. paprika
¼ tsp. chili powder
pinch onion powder
pinch cardamom
pinch garlic powder
pinch cinnamon
pinch ginger
Combine all spice ingredients in the small bowl, stir and set aside.

DIRECTIONS
Heat the olive oil in the saucepan. Add the onion and cook until soft, 2-3 minutes. Add the garlic, ginger, tomato and berbere seasoning and cook for 1-2 minutes. Add the salt, water and lentils and bring to a boil. Reduce heat to low, cover and simmer for 25-30 minutes (taste to make sure the lentils are soft – they may need an additional few minutes). Top with fresh cilantro and add salt if needed. Serve right away, or cool completely and refrigerate for up to 3 days.

PAN-ROASTED TOMATOES AND POLENTA

This polenta with mixed vegetables is a dish I crave over and over. Aside from eating it, my favorite part of this meal is the bursting of the tomatoes during preparation. It's so joyful! The sauce is light and flavorful and goes perfectly with the vegetables. This meal is wonderful to eat on the trail – and surprisingly, no fuss either. It's delicious to eat at room temperature, just bring along a fork and a cloth napkin and find a picturesque spot to enjoy your meal.

PREP TIME: 30 minutes
TOTAL TIME: 1 hour, 15 minutes
SERVES: 3

EQUIPMENT
Medium saucepan with lid
Large skillet
Medium mixing bowl
Cutting board
Chef's knife

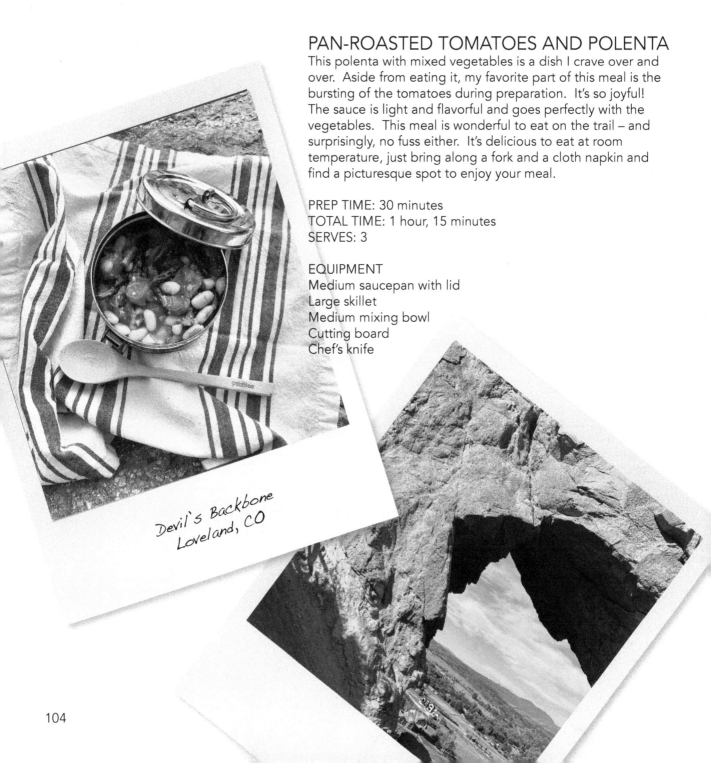

Devil's Backbone
Loveland, CO

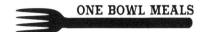

INGREDIENTS
3 ½ C. water
1 C. dry polenta
4 TBS. nondairy butter
½ tsp. salt
1 TBS. olive oil
¼ C. onion, diced
3-4 cloves of garlic, minced
2 serrano peppers, seeded and diced
2 tsp. ground cumin
2 C. cherry tomatoes
1 bunch of asparagus (about 10 medium-sized stalks), cut in 2" pieces
1 can northern beans, drained and rinsed
½ C. vegetable broth
Salt and pepper to taste
Nutritional yeast (optional)

DIRECTIONS
In the medium saucepan, add water and polenta. Stir then bring to a boil. Reduce heat to low and continue to cook, covered and stirring occasionally, for about 25-30 minutes. Near completion, add the butter and salt and stir. Turn off the heat/remove from heat source, cover and set aside until the rest of the meal is ready.

Add the oil to the skillet and when it's heated, add the onion and cook until soft, about 2-3 minutes. Add the garlic and peppers and cook for an additional 1-2 minutes. Stir in the cumin, then remove the pan from the burner. Put the cooked onion, garlic and peppers in the medium bowl and set aside. Place the skillet back on the burner (don't wash it!) on medium heat and add the tomatoes. Cook the tomatoes until they soften and their skin and juices begin to loosen. They might even pop or burst, adding a sizzle from their juices to the skillet. Add the onion/garlic/pepper mixture back to the skillet along with the asparagus, beans and broth. Bring to a boil, then reduce the heat to low and simmer for 10 minutes, uncovered. With the back of a fork, press gently on any tomatoes that didn't burst so all the juices get released.

If serving right away, place a generous scoop of the polenta on a large plate and spread into a circle. Ladle the tomato/asparagus mixture in the center. Top with a sprinkle of salt, pepper and nutritional yeast. Your meal can be stored in the refrigerator for up to 3 days. If taking out in nature, heat then place in an airtight container, then in an insulated bag.

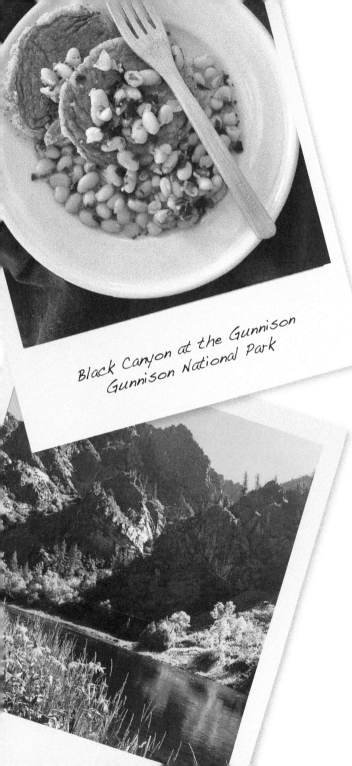

Black Canyon at the Gunnison
Gunnison National Park

BEANS, GREENS AND CORN CAKES

The beans and greens alone are a wonderful duo to satisfy your hunger, but when you add the corn cakes to the plate, they launch this meal to another place. There are many subtle flavors, yet the dish is simple to make and easy to enjoy – on the trail or at home. For the trail, pack the beans and greens mixture in an insulated container. In a separate container, pack the reheated corn cakes with a small square of parchment paper or wax paper in between each. To serve, pour the beans/greens over the corn cake and relish the savory goodness.

PREP TIME: 15 minutes
TOTAL TIME: 45 minutes
SERVES: 3

EQUIPMENT
Cutting board
Chef's knife
Large mixing bowl
Medium mixing bowl
Small mixing bowl
Large skillet
Spatula
Large plate or platter
Medium saucepan with lid

MAKE AHEAD The dry ingredients for the corncakes can put together in a bowl ahead of time and the greens can be chopped and refrigerated (for up to 2 days) until ready to use.

INGREDIENTS
2 TBS. olive oil
¼ tsp. mustard seeds
¼ tsp. cumin seeds
1 clove of garlic, minced
¼ C. onion, diced
1 small jalapeño (optional) diced with or without seeds

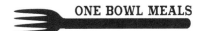

½ C. hearty greens, chopped (such as kale or collards)
1 C. vegetable broth
1 can of white beans (such as great northern or cannellini), rinsed
Salt and pepper to taste
Corn cakes (recipe below)

CORN CAKES
¾ C. all-purpose flour
¾ C. masa harina (cornflour)
2 TBS. sugar
2 tsp. baking powder
½ tsp. salt
¼ tsp. red pepper flakes
1 ¼ C. nondairy milk
Egg replacer (recipe below)
3 TBS. nondairy butter, melted
2 TBS. avocado or canola oil

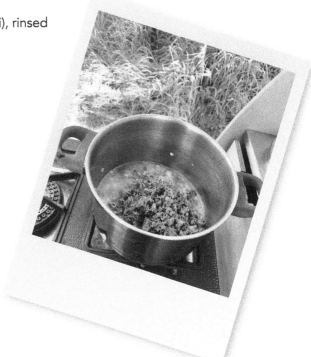

EGG REPLACER
1 TBS. ground flaxseed (also called flaxseed meal)
3 TBS. water
Put ingredients in the small bowl, stir and set aside.

CORN CAKES DIRECTIONS
In a large mixing bowl, add the dry ingredients (flour, cornflour, sugar, baking powder, salt, red pepper flakes) and stir. In a medium bowl, add the milk, egg replacer and butter. Stir until well blended. Add the wet ingredients to the dry ones and mix well. Heat the oil in the skillet. Ladle batter (enough for your pancake size preference) into the skillet. When golden brown, flip with the spatula and cook equally on the other side. Place cooked cakes on a large plate.

DIRECTIONS
In the medium saucepan, heat the olive oil on medium heat. Add the mustard and cumin seeds. Heat until they begin to pop, about 2 minutes. Add garlic, onion and jalapeño and cook until soft, about 2-3 minutes. Add greens then stir. Cook for an additional minute. Add broth and beans. Bring to a boil, cover, then turn the heat down to low. Simmer for 10 minutes then turn the heat off/remove from heat source. Taste and add salt if needed. If enjoying right away, plate 1-2 corncakes and ladle the beans/greens mixture on top. If storing for later, let both the beans/greens mixture and corn cakes cool completely, then store separately in the refrigerator for up to 3 days.

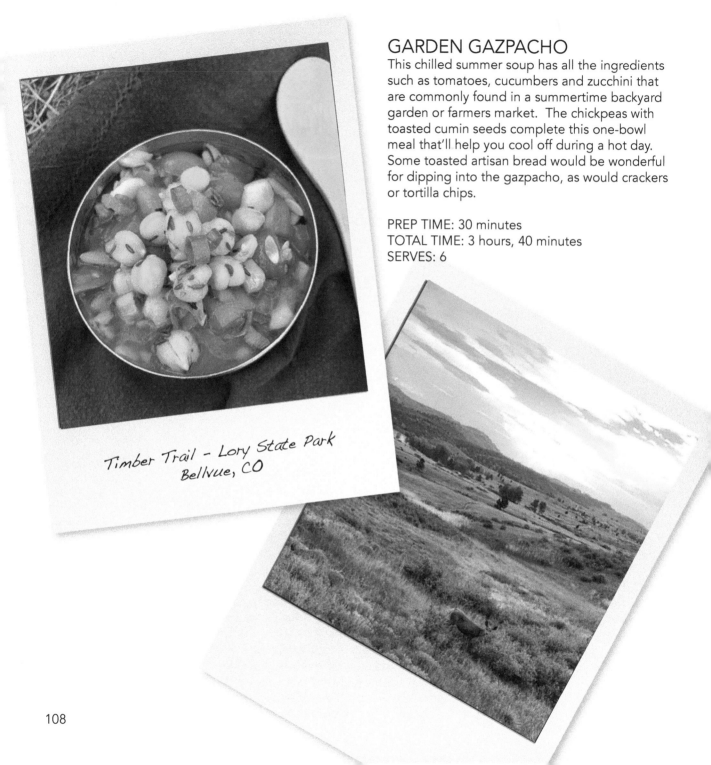

GARDEN GAZPACHO

This chilled summer soup has all the ingredients such as tomatoes, cucumbers and zucchini that are commonly found in a summertime backyard garden or farmers market. The chickpeas with toasted cumin seeds complete this one-bowl meal that'll help you cool off during a hot day. Some toasted artisan bread would be wonderful for dipping into the gazpacho, as would crackers or tortilla chips.

PREP TIME: 30 minutes
TOTAL TIME: 3 hours, 40 minutes
SERVES: 6

Timber Trail - Lory State Park
Bellvue, CO

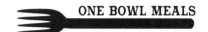
EQUIPMENT
Chef's knife
Cutting board
Large mixing bowl
Small frying pan
Kitchen towel
Medium mixing bowl

INGREDIENTS
6 C. fresh ripe tomatoes, diced
1 C. cucumber, chopped
1 C. zucchini, chopped
1 shallot, minced
½ C. olive oil
2 TBS. sherry vinegar
½ C. water
2 tsp. salt
Chickpeas with toasted cumin (recipe below)
3 green onions, sliced green parts for garnish

CHICKPEAS WITH TOASTED CUMIN
1 cans of chickpeas, rinsed and drained
1 TBS. olive oil
2 tsp. cumin seeds
Add the cumin seeds to the small frying pan over medium heat. Heat for 1-2 minutes, until slightly browned and fragrant. Turn off the heat and cool. While the cumin seeds are cooling, lay out the chickpeas on a clean kitchen towel and gently massage them to encourage the skins to come off. Put the shelled chickpeas in the medium bowl. Add the olive oil and toasted cumin seeds to the chickpeas and gently stir. Use right away, or cover and place in the refrigerator to store.

DIRECTIONS
In the large mixing bowl, mix together the tomatoes, cucumber, zucchini, shallot, olive oil, sherry vinegar, water and salt. Cover and place in the refrigerator until chilled completely, at least 3-4 hours. Taste and add salt if needed. Ladle the gazpacho into a bowl (or an insulated container if taking on a trail). Top with desired amount of the chickpeas with toasted cumin seeds and green onions.

MISO YOGA POT

This concoction of miso (a savory fermented paste from Japan), warming spices and cruciferous vegetables is a treat for your body and soul. The vegetables and beans listed are suggestions – they can be swapped out for what's in season or what you are craving. With the high liquid content, a tight-sealing insulated container is best for taking this out into nature – don't forget a spoon and a cloth napkin. I love to taste each spoonful slowly, appreciating the flavors and nutritional benefits of every bite.

PREP TIME: 20 minutes
TOTAL TIME: 35 minutes
SERVES: 3

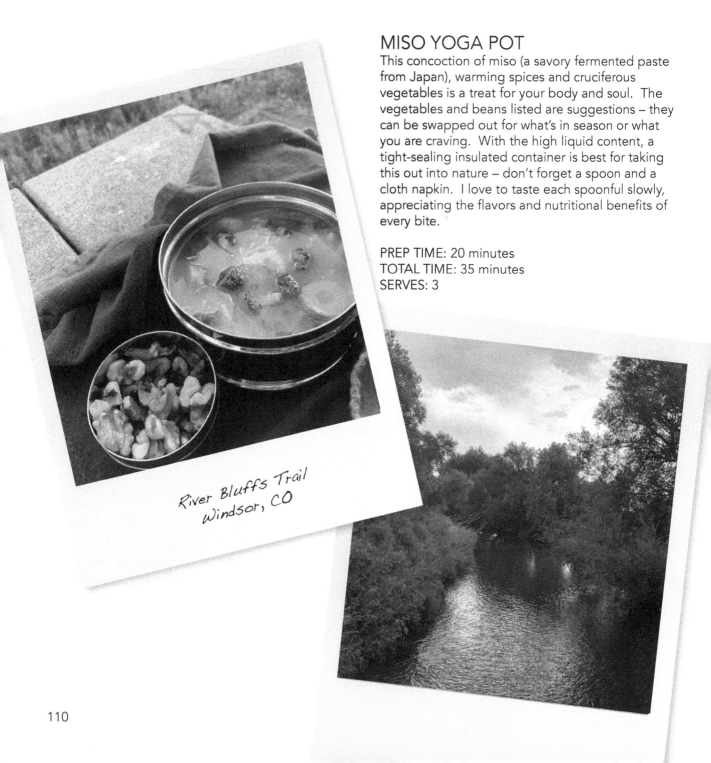

River Bluffs Trail
Windsor, CO

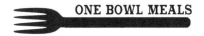

MAKE AHEAD: chopping the vegetables ahead of schedule (store in the refrigerator until ready to use) will make this already easy recipe even more simple!

EQUIPMENT
Chef's knife
Cutting board
Small mixing bowl
One large saucepan

INGREDIENTS
1 TBS. coconut oil
½ medium onion, diced
1" ginger, minced
3-4 cloves of garlic, minced
1 C. broccoli, cut into very small bite-sized pieces
1 C. cauliflower, cut into very small bite-sized pieces
1 C. kale, cut into very small bite-sized pieces
1 C. carrots, sliced thinly
1 C. leeks (white parts only), sliced thinly
2 TBS. white miso paste
4 C. water
Spice blend (recipe below)
1 15 oz. can of butter beans, drained and rinsed

SPICE BLEND
½ tsp. turmeric
½ tsp. salt
½ tsp. pepper
Pinch of cayenne (optional)
Pinch of cinnamon
Combine all spice blend ingredients in the small bowl, stir and set aside.

DIRECTIONS
In the saucepan add the coconut oil and turn the heat on medium. After the oil has melted, add the onion and cook for 2-3 minutes. Add the ginger and garlic and cook for another 1-2 minutes. Add the broccoli, cauliflower, kale, carrots, leeks, miso paste, water, spice blend and beans. Stir and bring to a boil, then reduce heat to low. Simmer uncovered for 15 minutes. Serve right away or cool completely and store in the refrigerator for up to 3 days.

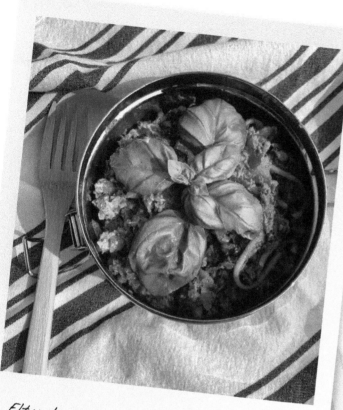

Eltuck Coves, Horsetooth Reservoir
Fort Collins, CO

VEGETABLE AND FRESH HERB PASTA BAKE

This amazing pasta bake is filled with your choice of vegetables, plus marinara sauce and creamy blended cashews. The walnuts in the sauce together with the sautéed vegetables mimic the heartiness of ground meat. I don't even bother reheating this dish when I head out for a hike – it's so easy to scoop into a container and get on your way!

PREP TIME: 35 minutes
TOTAL TIME: 55 minutes
SERVES: 6

MAKE AHEAD: Chop all the vegetables ahead of time and you'll be set to start cooking with minimal prep time when you're ready to make this meal.

EQUIPMENT
Large saucepan
Colander
Cutting board
Chef's knife
Large skillet with lid
9" x 12" baking dish (metal or glass)
Blender

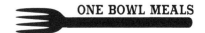

INGREDIENTS
5-6 quarts of water
Pinch of salt
1 box (1 lb.) of spaghetti
Creamed cashews (recipe below)
1 TBS. olive oil
½ medium onion, diced
5 C. chopped vegetable blend (such as zucchini, mushrooms, carrots, kale, peppers, etc.)
2 TBS. fresh oregano, chopped (or 1 tsp. dried)
2 TBS. fresh basil, chopped (or 1 tsp. dried)
1 C. walnuts, chopped
½ tsp. salt
½ tsp. pepper
¼ tsp. red pepper flakes
1 24 oz. jar of marinara sauce
½ tsp. salt
½ tsp. pepper
¼ tsp. red pepper flakes (optional)

CREAMED CASHEWS
1 C. raw cashews
1 C. hot water
Pinch of salt
Place ingredients in the blender (don't turn it on yet!) and let sit for 10 minutes. Then blend on high until completely smooth and creamy. Set aside.

DIRECTIONS
Preheat oven to 350 °. In the large saucepan bring the water and salt to a rolling boil. Add the spaghetti. Return to a boil, then reduce heat to low and simmer for 7-8 minutes, (until just under al dente – there will be more cooking time for the pasta in the oven), stirring occasionally. Drain in the colander then put in the baking pan. Pour the creamed cashews over the pasta (use a spoon to spread evenly) and set aside. Melt the oil in the skillet on medium heat. Add the onions and cook for 2-3 minutes. Add the chopped vegetables, herbs, walnuts, salt, pepper and red pepper flakes. Stir and cook (uncovered) for 5-7 minutes or until the vegetables are fork tender. Add the marinara sauce to the vegetable mixture, stir and turn off the heat/remove from heat source. Top the pasta with the marinara/vegetable mixture so that it covers the pasta with cashew cream completely. Place in the oven (uncovered) for 20 minutes. Let sit 5 minutes to cool down slightly then serve. Or cool completely and put in the refrigerator for up to 3 days. This freezes well to enjoy another time!

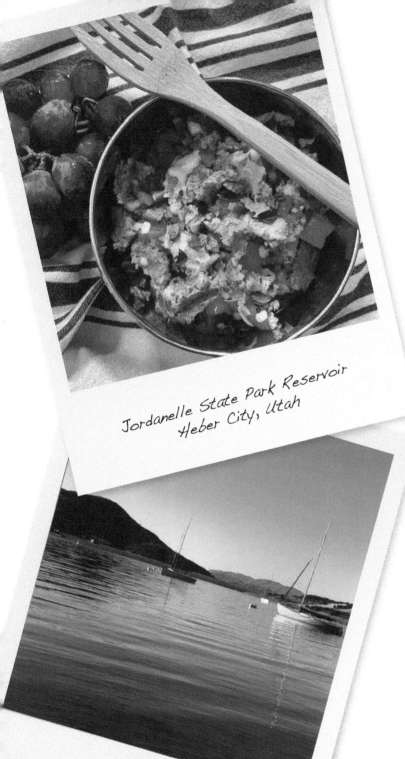

Jordanelle State Park Reservoir
Heber City, Utah

FALAFEL CRUMBLE BOWL

I love making this simple salad! Since the falafel patties are crumbled up, there's no need for perfection in the process. Just enjoy it – create an experience in the kitchen that's just as fun as you would on the trail. Pack up your salad in an airtight container and an insulated bag before heading out into the great outdoors for your hike.

PREP TIME: 25 minutes
TOTAL TIME: 2 hours 40 minutes (includes falafel mix advised refrigeration time)
SERVES: 4 (makes 8 patties (2 ¼" round)

MAKE AHEAD: The creamy tahini sauce can be made ahead and stored in the refrigerator for up to 3 days in advance.

EQUIPMENT
Food processor
Cutting board
Chef's knife
Spatula
Medium mixing bowl
Small mixing bowl
Whisk
Large skillet
Zester

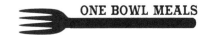

INGREDIENTS

1 15 oz. can of drained and rinsed chickpeas
¼ C. onion, diced
3-4 cloves of garlic
3 TBS. all-purpose flour
½ tsp. baking soda
½ C. plus 1 TBS. parsley, chopped and divided
1 TBS. sesame seeds

Spice blend (recipe below)
1 TBS. olive oil
Creamy tahini sauce (recipe below)
4 C. romaine lettuce, cut into bite-sized pieces
1 medium tomato, diced
Lemon zest from ½ a lemon

SPICE BLEND

¼ tsp. chili powder
½ tsp. cumin
Pinch of coriander
1 tsp. salt
Combine all spice blend ingredients in the small bowl, stir and set aside.

CREAMY TAHINI SAUCE

½ C. tahini
¼ C. water
¼ tsp. salt
In the medium mixing bowl, add the tahini, water and salt. Whisk until creamy and well blended. Set aside or store in an airtight container in the refrigerator, up to 3 days.

DIRECTIONS

In a food processor add the chickpeas, onion, garlic, flour, baking soda and ½ cup of the parsley and pulse until blended. Add the sesame seeds and spice blend and pulse a few more times. You may need to scrape down the mixture from the sides and pulse until blended. Transfer the mixture to a bowl and cover. Put in the fridge for 1-2 hours (you can skip this step – the mixture without refrigeration will be slightly more fragile, but still delicious). In the skillet, add the olive oil and turn the heat on medium. When the pan is heated add 2 tablespoons of the falafel mixture and press down with a spatula to flatten. Continue until the pan is filled and that there is enough space in between the falafels to flip them over when they are ready. When they start to get golden brown on the edges turn them over to cook evenly on the other side. Place the patties on a plate to cool. When cooled, use your fingers to gently crumble the patties. Divide the crumbles into 4 servings.

PLATING

Place the romaine lettuce at the bottom of the bowl. Add the tomatoes and falafel crumbles. Drizzle the creamy tahini dressing over your salad, then sprinkle the reserved parsley, lemon zest and a tiny pinch of salt on top.

SUPER SIMPLE BLACK BEAN SOUP

This one-pot meal is one of my staples – it has just a few ingredients and is easy to whip up in little time. The flavors from the spices make the beans and tomatoes shine. I like to toast a couple pieces of grainy bread to dip in the soup. Tortilla chips or crackers also pair well. On cooler days I heat it up, put it in an insulated container and take it out with me in nature – it makes for a belly-warming pit stop.

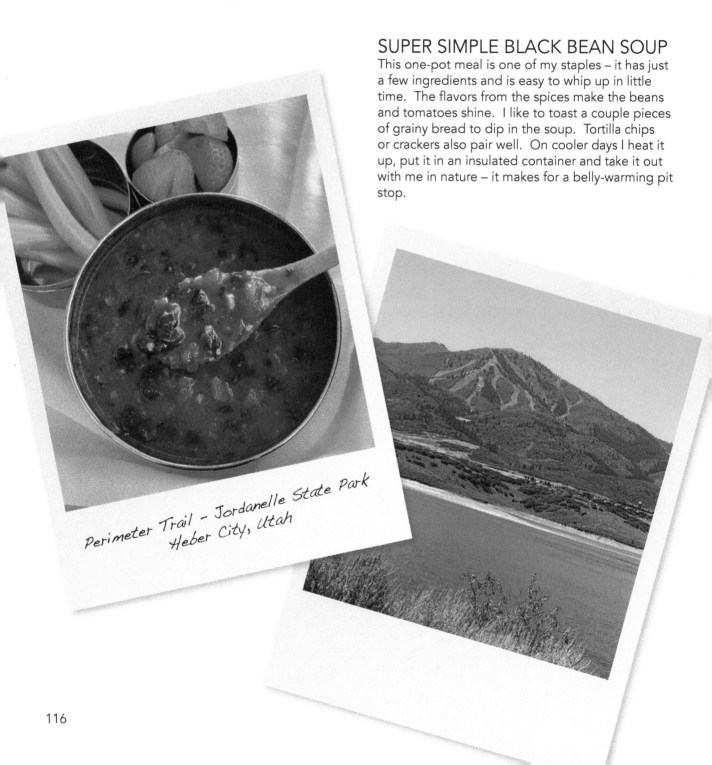

Perimeter Trail - Jordanelle State Park
Heber City, Utah

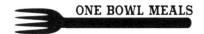

PREP TIME: 10 minutes
TOTAL TIME: 30 minutes
SERVES: 4-6

EQUIPMENT
Large saucepan
Colander
Chef's knife
Cutting board
Potato masher utensil
Small mixing bowl

INGREDIENTS
2 TBS. olive oil
½ onion, diced
1 jalapeño pepper (optional), with or without seeds, diced
3-4 cloves of garlic, minced
Spice blend (see recipe below)
4 C. vegetable broth
2 15 oz. cans of black beans, drained and rinsed
1 15 oz. can of fire-roasted diced tomatoes
Fresh cilantro, chopped

SPICE BLEND
½ tsp. salt
1 tsp. ground cumin
1 tsp. oregano
2 tsp. chili powder
Combine all spice blend ingredients in the small bowl, stir and set aside.

DIRECTIONS
Heat the olive oil in the saucepan on medium. Add the onion and cook for 2-3 minutes. Add the pepper and garlic and cook for 1-2 minutes. Add the spice blend and stir. Add the broth, beans and tomatoes. Bring to a boil then turn heat down to low and simmer for 10 minutes. Turn off heat/remove from heat source. Use the potato masher to mash down the beans and tomatoes until you have the consistency you desire. Ladle into a bowl and top with the freshly chopped cilantro. Enjoy your soup right away, or allow to cool completely and store in the refrigerator for up to 3 days. This also freezes well to enjoy another time.

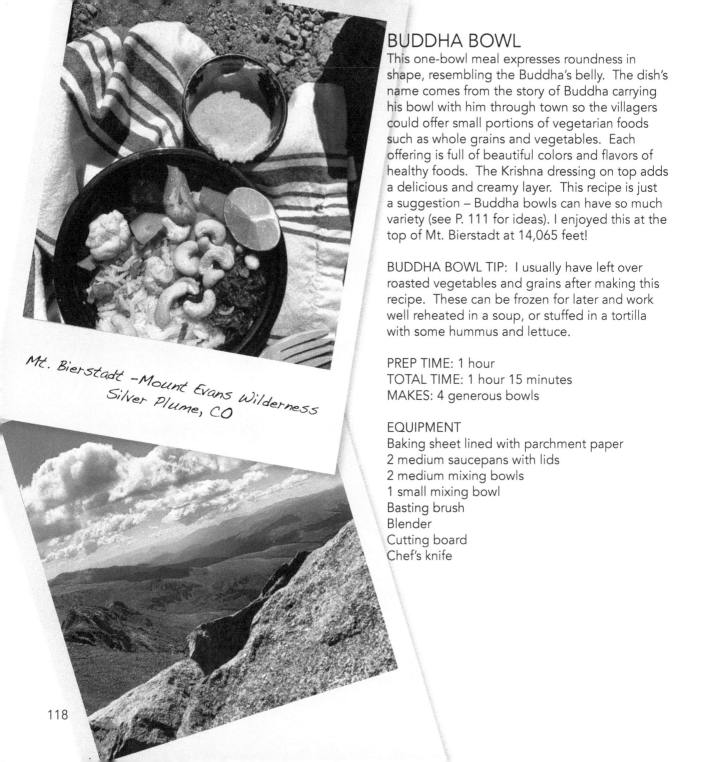

Mt. Bierstadt – Mount Evans Wilderness
Silver Plume, CO

BUDDHA BOWL

This one-bowl meal expresses roundness in shape, resembling the Buddha's belly. The dish's name comes from the story of Buddha carrying his bowl with him through town so the villagers could offer small portions of vegetarian foods such as whole grains and vegetables. Each offering is full of beautiful colors and flavors of healthy foods. The Krishna dressing on top adds a delicious and creamy layer. This recipe is just a suggestion – Buddha bowls can have so much variety (see P. 111 for ideas). I enjoyed this at the top of Mt. Bierstadt at 14,065 feet!

BUDDHA BOWL TIP: I usually have left over roasted vegetables and grains after making this recipe. These can be frozen for later and work well reheated in a soup, or stuffed in a tortilla with some hummus and lettuce.

PREP TIME: 1 hour
TOTAL TIME: 1 hour 15 minutes
MAKES: 4 generous bowls

EQUIPMENT
Baking sheet lined with parchment paper
2 medium saucepans with lids
2 medium mixing bowls
1 small mixing bowl
Basting brush
Blender
Cutting board
Chef's knife

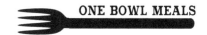

INGREDIENTS
Roasted vegetables (see recipe below)
½ C. brown or green lentils (see recipe below)
½ C. brown rice (see recipe below)
1 C. marinated kale, cut into very small bites (see recipe, next page)
1 C. nuts (such as cashews, almonds, or pecans)
Almond Krishna dressing (recipe, P. 122)

ROASTED VEGETABLES
Vegetables such as carrots, potatoes, cauliflower, broccoli, bell pepper, onion, asparagus, brussels
sprouts (enough to fill a baking sheet, cut any way that appeals to you)
2 TBS. olive oil
½ tsp. turmeric
½ tsp. salt
½ tsp. ground cumin
Peel (or don't) and trim your vegetables to your liking and place on the lined baking sheet. In the small
mixing bowl, add the olive oil, turmeric, salt and cumin and stir. Baste the vegetables generously until
all the oil and spices are gone. Bake for 30 minutes – check to see if they are fork tender (they may
need a couple extra minutes). Some vegetables may be cooked fully before the others. Remove the
fully cooked vegetables from the oven and give the rest extra time as needed. Set aside to cool. When
ready to plate, divide the bounty into four portions.

COOKED LENTILS
½ C. dry lentils
1 ½ C. vegetable broth or water
In the medium saucepan, bring lentils and water to a boil, then reduce heat, cover and simmer for 25
minutes. Check to see if the lentils are tender. They may need a few more minutes, but don't cook to
the point that they are mushy. When ready to plate, place ¼ C. of the lentils into the bowl.

COOKED BROWN RICE
½ C. dry brown rice
1 C. vegetable broth or water
¼ tsp. salt
In the medium saucepan, bring water, rice and salt to a boil, then reduce heat, cover and simmer for
40-45 minutes. Check at 40 minutes to see if the water has been absorbed. If not, place the lid back on
and cook for a few more minutes. When ready to plate, place ¼ C. of the rice into the bowl.

(Continued, next page)

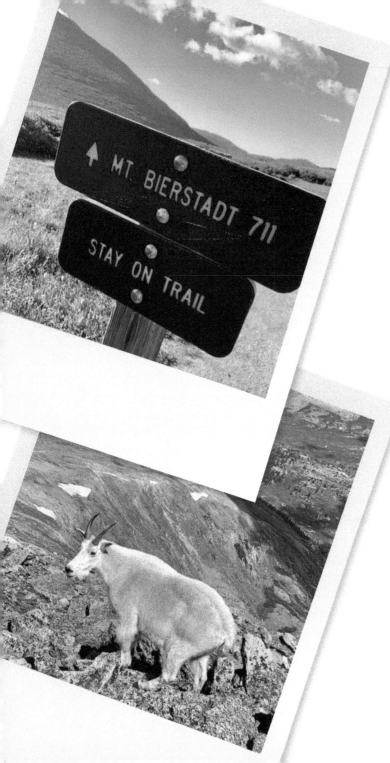

MARINATED KALE

2 C. kale, cut into very small bite-size pieces
¼ C. olive oil
Pinch of salt
Pinch of pepper

Place ingredients in the medium bowl and massage with your hands until everything is fully mixed together and the kale begins to break down. Place in the refrigerator, covered, to marinate for at least an hour. When ready to plate, place ¼ C. of the kale into the bowl.

ALMOND KRISHNA DRESSING

1 C. raw almonds
¼ C. avocado oil
1 C. water
2 TBS. liquid aminos (or soy sauce, or soy sauce alternative)
2 TBS. nutritional yeast
¼ tsp. asafetida* (also called hing – available online or at a specialty spice shop). To substitute hing/asafetida use ¼ tsp. onion powder plus ¼ tsp. garlic powder

Place all ingredients in the blender. Let the blender run at high speed for one minute. Remove the lid and check the consistency. If it is too thick, add more water. Store in the refrigerator for up to 3 days.

*Asafetida (or hing) is a flavor enhancing Indian spice – extracted from the roots of the Ferula plant. This spice offers anti-viral, anti-bacterial and anti-inflammatory properties.

BUILD YOUR BOWL

After adding the ¼ cup each of lentils, rice, kale, nuts and a serving of vegetables to your bowl, top it with the creamy Almond Krishna Dressing. Additional garnishes may include seeds or chopped fresh herbs.

ANATOMY OF A BUDDHA BOWL

Foods have such a big impact on our overall health and well-being. It is said that various foods contribute to balancing the chakras, or the major energy centers in our bodies. Our chakra systems represent our: need to belong (root), creativity (sacral), self-worth (solar plexus), capacity for love (heart), self expression (throat), focus (third eye) and universal connection (crown). Whether that resonates with you or not, we all agree that eating healthy foods contributes to healthy bodies.

BEANS/LEGUMES/TOFU
Edamame
Red, green, brown, black lentils
Chickpeas
Adzuki
Navy
Kidney
Black
Pinto
Blackeye
Great northern
Tofu/tempeh/
seitan

NUTS
Cashews
Almonds
Pistachio
Walnut
Macadamia
Peanut
Pine
Pecans

GREENS
Arugula
Watercress
Kale
Collard greens
Swiss chard/rainbow chard
Romaine
Spinach
Cilantro
Parsley
Mint

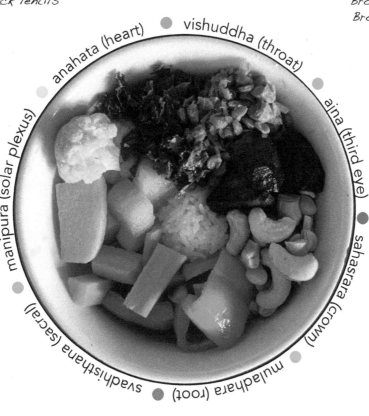

anahata (heart)
vishuddha (throat)
ajna (third eye)
manipura (solar plexus)
sahasrara (crown)
svadhisthana (sacral)
muladhara (root)

WHOLE GRAINS
Brown/white rice
Brown/white basmati rice
Brown/white jasmine rice
Wild rice
Barley
Farro
Millet

SEEDS
Quinoa (yes, a seed!)
Sunflower
Poppy
Hemp
Flax
Sesame
Pepitas

ROASTED VEGETABLES
Red peppers
Carrots
Yellow/white potatoes
Sweet potatoes
Cauliflower
Broccoli
Golden/purple beets
Brussles sprouts
Onion
Squash
Green beans
Tomatoes

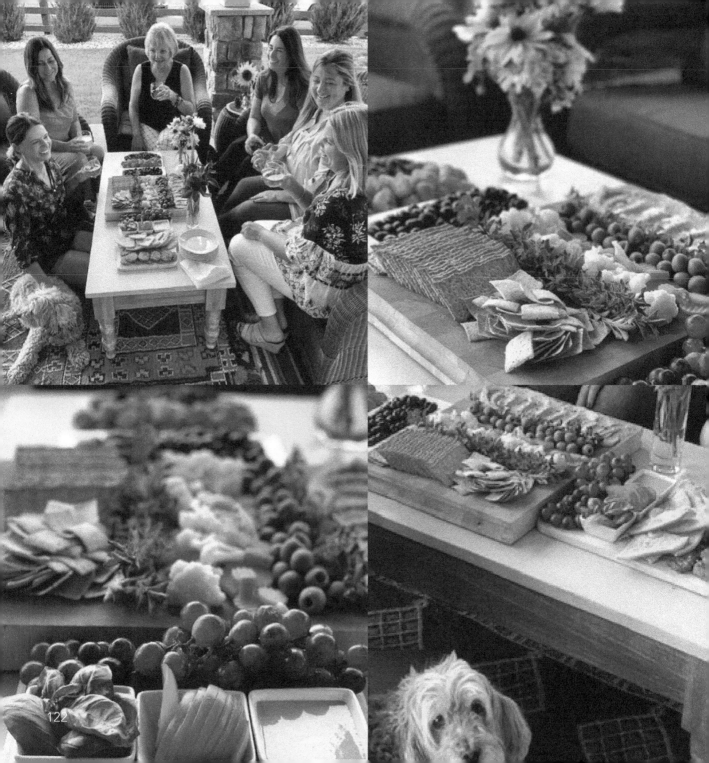

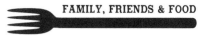

BUDDHA BOUNTY PARTY

A perfect plan for a party, this deconstructed Buddha bowl concept offers guests a variety of tempting options to gather around and nosh. Use a long serving platter or board (or many cutting boards side by side); arrange the food artistically, with no bounds, guided by your own imagination. It's casual, easy and fun for all to sit back, relax and unwind. You as the host can make all the food (plan for guests with dietary restrictions) – or if it's more of a potluck style event, have your friends each bring an assigned dish to contribute to the meal. The main priority is ease: This style of gathering can be planned just a few days ahead or even put together last minute. Your focus should be on family, friends, food and joy!

PLAN AHEAD
- Make a list of the items you want to serve (see suggestions below)
- Plan your grocery list and shop 2-3 days before your event date
- Clean the kitchen, dining area and bathroom 1-2 days in advance

INVITATION
Rally your guests by text, email, Evite or with a printed invitation at least a week in advance (when possible!).

MUSIC
Make a custom playlist or have a couple of radio stations in mind that play the music that reflects the general mood and theme of the occasion. A few ideas for tunes that might hit the spot: classical, nature sounds, Calypso, disco, show tunes or hits from your favorite decade.

CANDLES/LIGHTING
Candles add a lovely, celebratory feel, but remember: Guests should smell the food – not the candle – so be sure to use unscented candles at your event. Small votive candles or tealights in pretty cups look beautiful sprinkled throughout the space.

FRESH FLOWERS
Flowers are always a nice touch if you have room on your table or in the general area of your event. Small bud vases spread throughout work well to add color and won't overwhelm the space as one large arrangement might (unless you have a space that works!).

DRINKS
If you'll be serving alcoholic beverages, consider choosing simple white and red wines that have wide appeal, and/or creating a single unique, original cocktail especially for your event. Be sure to have nonalcoholic choices on hand as well. Fresh garnishes like lime/lemon wedges, edible flowers and herb fronds are festive and make whatever drink your guest chooses extra special.

DAY OF EVENT
Set up plates, napkins, utensils, glasses, food platters/boards, beverage area, candle and flower locations.

Toasted cashews   Pickled vegetables   Stuffed mushrooms   Olives   White bean dip   Hummus   Black bean and corn salsa   Guacamole   Fresh tomato salsa   Crackers   Tortilla chips   Mini roasted vegetable skewers   Corn fritters   Roasted almonds   Walnuts   Baked kale   Baguette slices   Fresh-cut carrots   Marinated artichokes   Tomato slices with fresh herbs   Baked sweet potato slices   Baked zucchini chips   Roasted broccoli   Vegetable fritters   Sliced cucumber   Oven-baked potato wedges   Roasted cauliflower   Avocado slices   Marinated kale   Falafel patties with mini pita bread rounds   Bell pepper slices   Crispy chickpeas   Orange slices   Mango slices   Apple slices with cinnamon   Grapes   Dark chocolate bark   Dark chocolate covered pretzels   Dark chocolate covered almonds   Candied pecans   Truffles   Mini muffins   Dessert breads

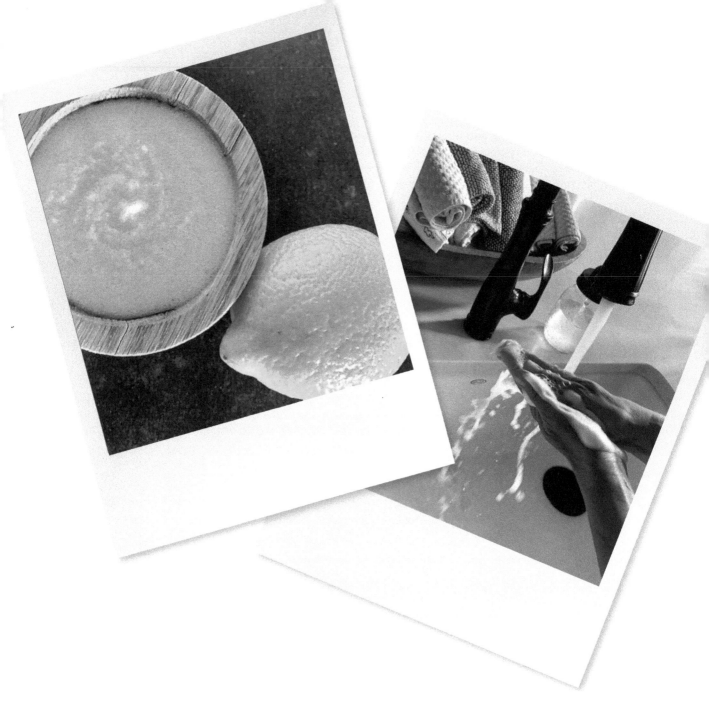

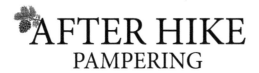

AFTER HIKE
PAMPERING

COCONUT SUGAR SCRUB

After your hike you are probably due for a shower! Take this scrub with you into the bath or shower – it both exfoliates and moisturizes your skin. The essential oil combination below is just a personal favorite of mine – you may have other oil(s) you prefer to use. There are endless combinations and options (for example, try lavender and rosemary for a calming scent). The scrub makes a great gift, too. Your hands and feet will be especially thankful! Scrub and glow!

PREP TIME: 10 minutes
TOTAL TIME: 15 minutes
MAKES: 4 ½ cups

EQUIPMENT
Countertop kitchen mixer (or large bowl if done by hand)
Rubber spatula
Glass or recycled plastic containers for coconut scrub

INGREDIENTS
3 C. sugar
1 ½ C. coconut oil
½ tsp. lemon essential oil
½ tsp. peppermint essential oil
1 tsp. vitamin e oil (optional)

DIRECTIONS
In the countertop mixer bowl (or large bowl), add all the ingredients. Turn on low or mix by hand for 1-2 minutes until well combined – don't over-blend, though, as the sugar could melt. Use the rubber spatula to guide the scrub into your container(s). Store in a cool place that doesn't get sunlight.

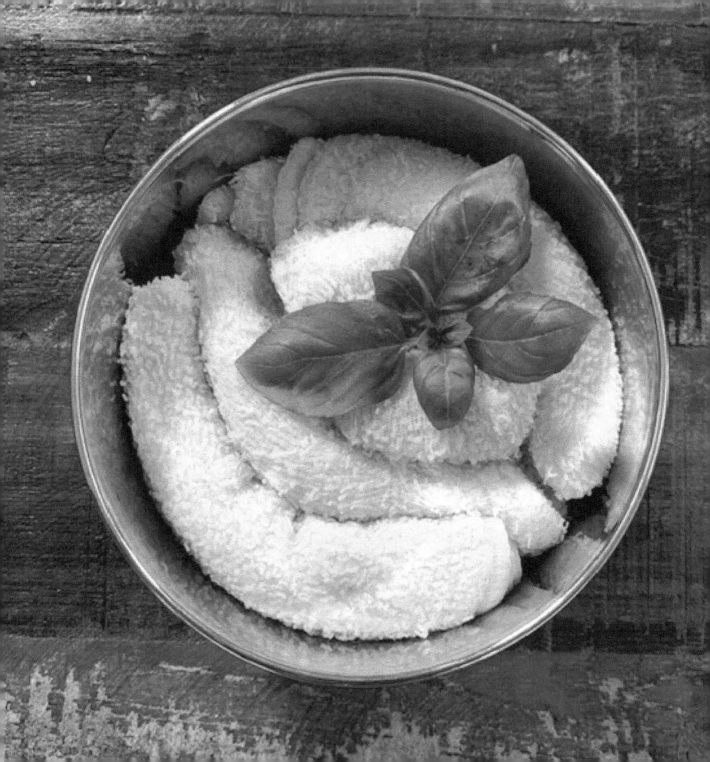

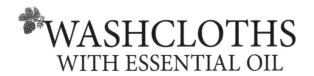# WASHCLOTHS
WITH ESSENTIAL OIL

SUPPLIES
4 clean washcloths
Large mixing bowel
Water
Essential oil

DIRECTIONS
Place the washcloths in the mixing bowl and fill with water until the cloths are submerged. Add 8-10 drops of essential oil. One washcloth at a time, squeeze out the excess water and fold in half, then roll it up tightly from the short side. Place in a leak-proof container or freezer bag and put in the freezer. If taking the washcloths on the trail, keep them in the freezer bag and place in an insulated bag for your backpack so they're cool and refreshing when you use them.

Here are some of my go-to essential oils individually or as a blend:

- eucalyptus
- peppermint
- spearmint
- pine needle
- lavender
- sandalwood
- citronella
- cypress
- geranium
- grapefruit
- lemon
- lime
- rosemary

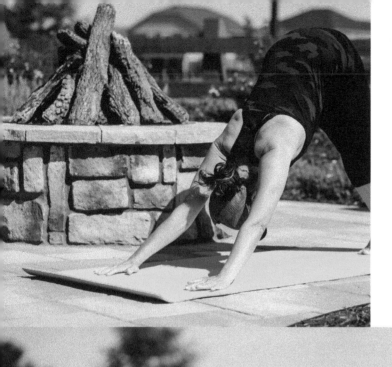

7 POSES, 5 BREATHS EACH

This short yoga posture sequence stretches the shoulders, opens the side body, stretches the hamstrings, lengthens the spine, opens the hips, and strengthens the low back. Your mind is offered a break to be cleared and centered from everyday distractions. Your spirit will be refreshed and renewed. In ten short minutes this sequence offers increased strength and flexibility, promotes circulatory health, reduces anxiety and increases energy and vitality.

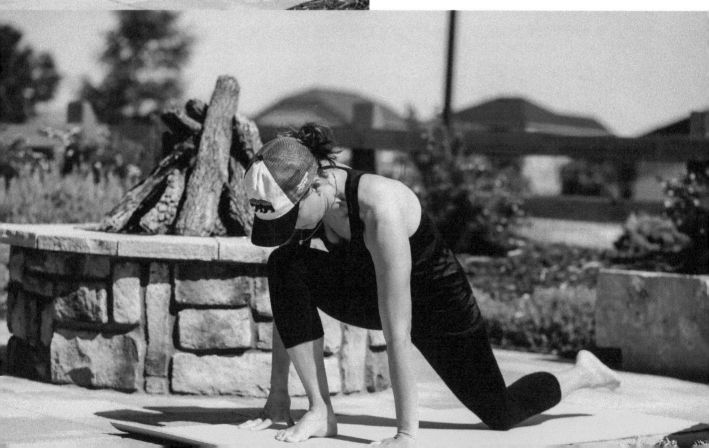

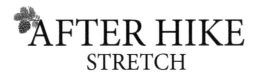

AFTER HIKE
STRETCH

10 MINUTE AFTER HIKE YOGA SEQUENCE

MOUNTAIN POSE Begin standing tall. Press the feet into the earth and center yourself. Steady the breath and clear the mind. Stay for five full rounds of breath.

UPWARD SALUTE POSE From Mountain Pose – inhale and raise the arms overhead and reach high until the palms come together. On the exhale, draw the palms downward to your heart center. Stay for five full rounds of breath.

SIDE BEND Raise the left arm up to the sky, the right arm extends down by your side. The left arm reaches up even more, then over to the right; the right arm extends long, your right hand reaches down towards your right ankle. This will open the left side body. Keep the feet pressed firmly into the earth. Now do the right side. Stay for five full rounds of breath on each side.

FORWARD FOLD From standing, raise both arms up overhead on the inhale. On the exhale gently begin to fold your upper body towards the ground. Bend your knees as much as you need as you hinge at the hips. Adjust your feet position as needed and grab opposite elbows or upper arms with your hands. Let the upper body hang, keeping the head heavy and neck very loose and soft. You have the option to sway slightly from side to side if the movement feels good. Stay for five breaths. Release the hands to the earth, keeping the body in a forward fold position.

LOW LUNGE From the forward fold, step the right leg back (hands on the earth framing the left foot to stay steady). Keep the hands on the ground or raise them up to the sky (your knee can come down to the mat for more stability or can be lifted for a deeper stretch). Let the hips melt towards the earth. Stay for five breaths. Now do the left side.

LOCUST Come down to your belly, forehead and hips pressed to the floor or mat. Squeeze the legs towards each other. Interlace the fingers behind your back (or, if your hands don't connect, use a towel, belt or strap held in both hands to make this more accessible). Lift the head, chest, arms and feet. Stay for five breaths. On the final exhale, release the body completely back to the earth.

DOWNWARD FACING DOG From the belly down, bend the knees and tuck the toes under. On the next inhale press your hands into the earth and raise the hips up high, keeping the knees bent as much as you need, or straightening them all the way. Stay for five breaths. Finish the sequence by walking the feet towards the hands (you will be in a forward fold). On the next inhale, guide the torso upright into a standing position with the arms raised upwards and the palms drawn together. On the exhale draw the palms to your heart center. Experience gratitude and smile.

OM LOKAH SAMASTHA SUKHINO BHAVANTU
- MAY ALL BEINGS BE HEALTHY, HAPPY AND FREE -

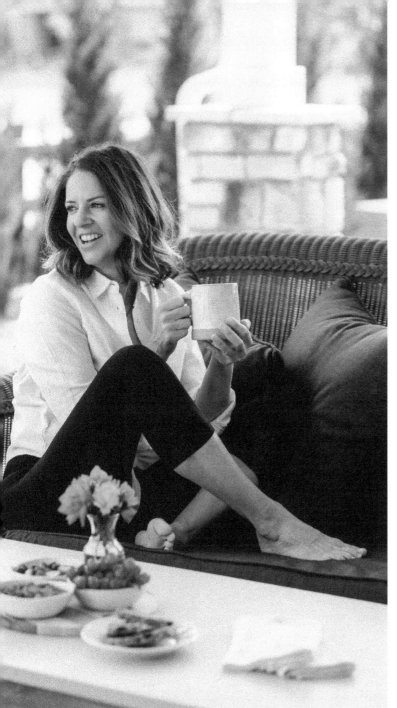

ABOUT THE AUTHOR

Marty is a self-proclaimed master of fun, who loves to rally the troops to hit the trail, gawk over the gorgeous scenery and eat some great home-made food along the way. She has been known to talk first-time hikers into headlamps and a 3am departure for the adventure and promise of a stunning mountain sunrise.*

A certified yoga teacher, she credits her daily yoga, meditation practice and 10+ years of a plant-based lifestyle to keep her centered, strong and limber for the next hike. Whether it is a 14,000'+ peak or a smooth and easy trail, she embraces all hikes with the joy of the opportunity to explore nature.

Marty lives with her husband, their two rowdy teenage boys and two rowdy dogs (also boys) in Fort Collins, Colorado. She wouldn't have it any other way.

The next adventure in nature awaits!
Trek to tabletotrail.com

*They only agreed because she promised to schlep her oven baked granola, oat milk and serve hot tea at the summit.

CPSIA information can be obtained
at www.ICGtesting.com
Printed in the USA
LVHW010938251120
672647LV00003B/37

9 780578 728445